ABC of
Neurodevelopmental Disorders

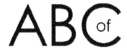

ABC of

Neurodevelopmental Disorders

Edited by

Munib Haroon

Consultant Community Paediatrician & Trust Lead for Paediatric ADHD
Pinderfields Hospital
Mid Yorkshire Teaching NHS Trust
Wakefield, UK

WILEY Blackwell

Registered Offices
John Wiley & Sons, Inc., 111 River Street, Hoboken, NJ 07030, USA
John Wiley & Sons Ltd, The Atrium, Southern Gate, Chichester, West Sussex, PO19 8SQ, UK

For details of our global editorial offices, customer services, and more information about Wiley products visit us at www.wiley.com.

Wiley also publishes its books in a variety of electronic formats and by print-on-demand. Some content that appears in standard print versions of this book may not be available in other formats.

Library of Congress Cataloging-in-Publication Data
Names: Haroon, Munib, editor.
Title: ABC of neurodevelopmental disorders / [edited by] Munib Haroon.
Description: Hoboken, NJ : Wiley-Blackwell, 2024. | Includes index.
Identifiers: LCCN 2023054312 (print) | LCCN 2023054313 (ebook) | ISBN
    9781119900177 (paperback) | ISBN 9781119900184 (adobe pdf) | ISBN
    9781119900153 (epub)
Subjects: MESH: Neurodevelopmental Disorders
Classification: LCC RJ486.5 (print) | LCC RJ486.5 (ebook) | NLM WS 350.7
    | DDC 618.92/8–dc23/eng/20240112
LC record available at https://lccn.loc.gov/2023054312
LC ebook record available at https://lccn.loc.gov/2023054313

Cover Design by Wiley
Cover Image: © iMrSquid/Getty Images

Set in 9.25/12pt Minion by Straive, Pondicherry, India

SKY10065936_012424

Contents

List of Contributors

Julie Armstrong
SEND Development Team Manager
Wakefield Council
Wakefield, UK

Elizabeth Birley
Specialty Doctor, Community Paediatrics
Hull University Teaching Hospitals NHS Trust
Hull, UK

Conor Davidson
Consultant Psychiatrist
Clinical Lead, Leeds Autism Diagnostic Service
Royal College of Psychiatrists Autism Champion
Leeds, UK

Sharmi Ghosh
Higher Trainee in Psychiatry
Leeds Autism Diagnostic Service
Leeds, UK

Munib Haroon
Consultant Community Paediatrician & Trust Lead for Paediatric ADHD
Pinderfields Hospital
Mid Yorkshire Teaching NHS Trust
Wakefield, UK

Alwyn Kam
Specialty Doctor in Psychiatry of Learning Disability
Leeds Autism Diagnostic Service
Leeds, UK

Tracy Laverick
Senior Educational Psychologist and Lecturer
Leeds Trinity University
Leeds, UK

Keri-Michèle Lodge
Consultant in the Psychiatry of Intellectual Disability
Leeds and York Partnership NHS Foundation Trust
Leeds, UK

Mini Pillay
Consultant Child and Adolescent Psychiatrist (Learning Disabilities)
Rotherham Doncaster and South Humber NHS Foundation Trust
Rotherham, UK

Ayesha Qureshi
Consultant Community Paediatrician
Allens Croft Children's Centre
Birmingham Community Healthcare Trust
Birmingham, UK

F. Lucy Raymond
Professor of Medical Genetics and Neurodevelopment
Department of Medical Genetics
University of Cambridge
Cambridge, UK

Fraser Scott
Paediatric Consultant & Trust Lead for Paediatric Epilepsy
Pinderfields Hospital
Mid Yorkshire Teaching NHS Trust
Wakefield, UK

Monica Shaha
CAMHS Clinical Lead
Psychiatry-UK LLP
Leeds, UK

Preface

Unlike the contributors to this book, the vast majority of healthcare professionals are not in the business of diagnosing and/or managing neurodevelopmental conditions (or 'disorders', to use the official nomenclature). But it is highly likely, given the prevalence of such disorders, that the typical doctor, nurse, therapist or equivalent will be involved in the care of people who are neurodivergent at some point in their career. As such, I have always believed that learning about neurodiversity and the conditions/disorders frequently associated with such states of being should get ample coverage in training and in continuing professional development programmes. Thus appropriate sources of information for professionals need to exist to support this (and also to help inform the interested person). These should not be so big as to be unwieldy, nor so small as to be almost uninformative. I hope this book straddles that Goldilocks zone, is easily digestible, and bears the reader in good stead for their clinical practice.

Munib Haroon

Acknowledgements

A very big 'thank you!' to all the chapter contributors and to your families and loved ones. I appreciate the time, dedication and expertise that has gone into the writing.

All the authors have learnt a lot from colleagues and mentors over the years, and also our patients – and this book has benefited from the collective experiences of interacting with them.

Thank you to Wiley for supporting another one of my endeavours. Starting with James Watson, the Commissioning Editor at the outset; Moyuri Handique, Managing Editor; and thank you also to Ella Elliot, Editorial Assistant. Thank you to Sally Osborn for your copyediting expertise and also Samras Johnson V, Content Refinement Specialist.

Thank you to Sarah Hughes, Laura Archer, Rebecca Barrass and Rachel Beanland for reading chapters and for making helpful suggestions. Thank you to Alison Stansfield for the use of work from our previous joint venture.

I would like to acknowledge the moral support of the Mid Yorkshire Teaching NHS Trust during the writing of this book, specifically Kath, Andrew, Denise, Freya, my departmental colleagues, and also the staff at the medical library, who have found papers at short notice, performed searches and helped obtain new books – and kept them checked out for me – and whose stock of fiction has also offered relief. I am grateful for the presence of the British Library in Boston Spa, a blessing to have such a great facility so far outside of London!

I want to thank a number of neurodivergent people (and their partners) who wrote some of the case studies. Thank you to M and N, and to Rizwan Iqbal for sharing your insights with me and with the future readership of this book. I am very grateful! Thank you also to Elizaveta Dydykina for writing a vignette, for reading and commenting on several chapters, providing suggestions for the cover image, and for sharing your thoughts about neurodiversity (and your encyclopaedic knowledge) with me; your thoughts have influenced my thinking and outlook, and this book is all the better for them.

Finally, my love and thanks to my family for their enduring support. A few short lines of thanks do not do justice to all the patience needed to put up with me, especially when I'm in 'writer's mode'. Thank you to HPPJ, for specific help with one section and for all the regular SMS messages. And to Malcolm, Carole, The Walkers, Abbo, Ammi, Sophie ('with the highest distinction') and Mubin: Thank you!

Munib Haroon
July 2023
North Yorkshire

Contributor Acknowledgements

For William, Sophie and Alice. You are my world. And for Andy, because he said I had to.

Elizabeth Birley

For my brother, David, and my father, Peter – brightest stars, you showed me the way. Shine on.

Keri-Michèle Lodge

For my mum, who would have been proud to see her son a published author but would have enjoyed correcting my English!

Fraser Scott

List of Abbreviations

3DI	Developmental, Dimensional and Diagnostic Interview
ADHD	attention deficit hyperactivity disorder
ADI-R	Autism Diagnostic Interview–Revised
ADL	activities of daily living
ADOS	Autism Diagnostic Observation Schedule
AHC	alternating hemiplegia of childhood
ARBD	alcohol-related birth defects
ARFID	avoidant restrictive food intake disorder
ARND	alcohol-related neurodevelopmental disorder
ASD	autism spectrum disorder
BACD	British Association of Childhood Disability
BARD	bipolar and related disorders
BAS 3	British Ability Scale 3
BDI	Beck Depression Inventory
BNF	British National Formulary
BOT-2	Bruininks-Oseretsky Test of Motor Proficiency Second Edition
BRIEF	Behavior Rating Inventory of Executive Function
CAMHS	Child and Adolescent Mental Health Services
CbD	cannabidiol
CBiT	comprehensive behavioural intervention for tics
CBT	cognitive behavioural therapy
CD	conduct disorder
CELF-5	Clinical Evaluation of Language Fundamentals–5
CGH	comparative genomic hybridisation
ChOCI	Obsessional Compulsive Inventory
CI	confidence interval
CNV	copy number variant
CSTS	cortico-striatal-thalamo-cortical
CTOPP-2	Comprehensive Test of Phonological Processing–2
DBS	deep brain stimulation
DBT	dialectical behaviour therapy
DCD	developmental coordination disorder
DEE	developmental and epileptic encephalopathy
DISCO	Diagnostic Interview for Social and Communication Disorders
DRPLA	dentatorubral-pallidoluysian atrophy
DSM-5-TR	*Diagnostic and Statistical Manual of Mental Disorders, Fifth Edition, Text Revision*
DSQIID	Dementia Screening Questionnaire for Individuals with Intellectual Disabilities
DVLA	Driver and Vehicle Licensing Agency
ECG	electrocardiogram
EDE-Q	Eating Disorder Examination Questionnaire
EEG	electroencephalogram
EHCP	Education, Health and Care plan
ERP	exposure and response prevention
EuPD	emotionally unstable personality disorder
FAS	foetal alcohol syndrome
FASD	foetal alcohol spectrum disorder
FHM	familial hemiplegic migraine
FMD	functional movement disorder
FND	functional neurological disorder
FTLB	functional tic-like behaviour
GARS-3	Gilliam Autism Rating Scale
GDD	global developmental delay
GORT-5	Grey Oral Reading Test–5
GWAS	genome-wide association study
HADS	Hospital Anxiety and Depression Scale
HCPC	Health and Care Professions Council
HIV	human immunodeficiency virus
HR	hazard ratio
HRT	habit reversal training
ICD	International Classification of Diseases
ID	intellectual disability
IDD	intellectual developmental disorder
IQ	intelligence quotient
LD	learning disability
MABC-2	Movement Assessment Battery for Children–Second Edition
MEP	motor evoked potential
MMR	measles, mumps and rubella
MRI	magnetic resonance imaging
MRR	mortality rate ratio
NBIA	neurodegeneration with brain iron accumulation
NDD	neurodevelopmental disorder
ND-PAE	neurobehavioural disorder associated with pre-natal alcohol exposure
NICE	National Institute for Health and Care Excellence
NMS	neuroleptic malignant syndrome

NSSI	non-suicidal self-injury	SD	standard deviation
OCD	obsessive compulsive disorder	SDQ	Strengths and Difficulties Questionnaire
OCI	Obsessive-Compulsive Inventory	SEN	special educational needs
ODD	oppositional defiant disorder	SENCO	special educational needs coordinator
OR	odds ratio	SIGN	Scottish Intercollegiate Guidelines Network
PAE	pre-natal alcohol exposure	SLD	specific learning difficulty
PANDAS	paediatric autoimmune neuropsychiatric disorder associated with streptococcal infection	SNAP	Swanson, Nolan and Pelham scale
PANS	paediatric acute-onset neuropsychiatric syndrome	SNP	single-nucleotide polymorphism
PANSS	Positive and Negative Syndrome Scale	SNRI	selective noradrenaline reuptake inhibitor
PDA	pathological demand avoidance	SpLD	specific learning disorder
PDD-NOS	pervasive developmental disorder not otherwise specified	SSRI	selective serotonin reuptake inhibitor
		STEEEP	safe, timely, effective, efficient, equitable, patient-centred
PEACE	Pathway for Eating disorders and Autism developed from Clinical Experience	STOMP	Stopping Over-Medication of People with a learning disability, autism or both
PED	paroxysmal exercise-induced dyskenesia	STAMP	Supporting Treatment and Appropriate Medication in Paediatrics
PF	palpebral fissure	SUD	substance use disorder
pFAS	partial foetal alcohol syndrome	SUDIC	sudden unexpected death in childhood
PhAB	Phonological Assessment Battery	TBS	theta burst stimulation
PKD	paroxysmal kinesiogenic dyskenesia	tDCS	transcranial direct current stimulation
PMD	paroxysmal movement disorder	THC	tetrahydrocannabinol
PNKD	paroxysmal non-kinesiogenic dyskenesia	TMS	transcranial magnetic stimulation
PRS	polygenic risk score	VOUS	variants of uncertain significance
PUTS	Premonitory Urge for Tics Scale	WIAT	Wechsler Individual Achievement Test
QbTest	Quantitative Behavioural Test	WISC	Wechsler Intelligence Scale for Children
RCADS	Revised Child Anxiety and Depression Scale	YARC	York Assessment of Reading Comprehension
RCT	randomised controlled trial	Y-BOCS	Yale Brown Obsessive-Compulsive Scale
rTMS	repetitive transcranial magnetic stimulation	YGTSS	Yale Global Tic Severity Scale
SASC	Specialist Assessments Standards Committee		

CHAPTER 1

An Introduction to Neurodevelopmental Disorders

Munib Haroon

OVERVIEW

- Neurodevelopmental disorders (NDDs) are relatively common conditions.
- They arise in the developing brain and so have features typically present in childhood.
- They can present with developmental differences and alterations in personal, social, academic or occupational functioning.
- They include autism, ADHD, Tourette's disorder/tic disorders, developmental coordination disorder, intellectual developmental disorders (intellectual disability) and specific learning disorder.
- NDDs often co-occur in the same individual.
- NDDs are associated with mental health difficulties and other physical conditions.
- NDDs can be viewed as diversity/difference/divergence, difficulty, disorders or disabilities, according to context and different models of health.

What is a neurodevelopmental disorder?

Neurodevelopmental disorders (see Box 1.1) arise in the developing brain; their features are typically present from childhood (but may escape attention until later on in adolescence or adulthood). They may include differences in patterns of development or result in alterations in personal, social, academic or occupational functioning.

Depending on the person and their situation, these conditions may be considered as natural (neuro) diversity, difference, neurodivergency and/or as difficulties, disorders or disabilities (see Box 1.1). There is typically a strong genetic component behind them, meaning that they can cluster in families. In addition, they often seem to co-occur in the same individual.

Classification schemes

Two of the main classification schemes in healthcare, the International Classification of Diseases (ICD) and the *Diagnostic and Statistical Manual of Mental Disorders* (DSM) (see Figure 1.1),

define what conditions are classed as neurodevelopmental disorders. Both of these are well-established, internationally recognised systems and at the time of writing are in their 11th and 5th iterations, plus further text revisions for the latter. While they continue to use slightly different terminology for some conditions, they have become more closely aligned over the years. This is helpful in ensuring the use of consistent terms. That is important, because consistent language can be helpful for clinicians who make diagnoses, but also for researchers, patients, carers and other professionals.

Table 1.1 lists some of the conditions classed as neurodevelopmental disorders; as you can see, the lists under each classification are very similar. Because the DSM is probably the most widely used system and the one that most people are familiar with, this book will use the DSM terminology.

Even after taking account of the conditions deliberately left out of the list in Table 1.1 for simplicity, there do seem to be some notable omissions. Tic disorders do not appear primarily under the ICD-11 classification, but instead appear as a secondary class. There are other conditions that could be said to belong in the classification schemes for neurodevelopmental conditions but are not listed. Examples include epilepsy and schizophrenia. Compelling arguments could be made for including these on the lists, although clearly counter-arguments against locating them there have also been made – and for the moment seem to dominate the discussion.

This demonstrates the somewhat arbitrary nature of classification schemes.

There are other conditions that will be familiar to some people as neurodevelopmental disorders but are not on these lists, for example Asperger's syndrome (see Box 1.2). This illustrates the changing nature of classification schemes. For example, conditions like Asperger's or 'pervasive developmental disorder not otherwise specified' have become subsumed within the more overarching term 'autism spectrum disorder'. There are a number of reasons for this; perhaps the most important is that many conditions are increasingly described as existing on a continuum, with variations in the extent to which individuals with these conditions manifest

ABC of Neurodevelopmental Disorders, First Edition. Edited by Munib Haroon.
© 2024 John Wiley & Sons Ltd. Published 2024 by John Wiley & Sons Ltd.

Box 1.1 **Some definitions**

A number of different terms are used throughout this text, such as condition, disorder, disability, neurodiversity, neurodivergent and neurotypical, of which brief definitions are given here. The reader should be aware that there may be variations in how these are used outside of this text.

- *Condition*: A general or specific state of physical/mental health (i.e. 'you're a highly conditioned athlete' vs 'the condition you have is called eczema'). In *ABC of Neurodevelopmental Disorders* the word is therefore frequently used to imply a variation from the 'usual' and sometimes in relation to a specific condition.
- *Disorder*: A condition or illness that affects the usual functioning of the body or mind.
- *Disability*: A physical or mental condition that has a substantial and long-term negative effect on the ability to do normal daily activities.
- *Neurodiversity*: The thinking, perceiving, learning and behavioural variations that exist across all humans (e.g. 'Neurodiversity is a fact of life' but *not* 'I am neurodiverse').
- *Neurodivergent*: The presence of variations from 'the norm' in thinking/perceive/learning/behaving (e.g. 'I am neurodivergent').
- *Neurotypical*: As distinct from neurodivergent. The type of thinking/perceiving/learning/behaving that conforms to what is understood to be 'usual' by society and does not fit a recognised pattern of thinking that might be identified as neurodivergent.

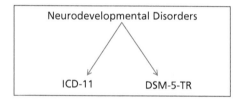

Figure 1.1 The classification schemes for neurodevelopmental disorders.

Table 1.1 Comparison of classification schemes ICD-11 and DSM-5-TR for neurodevelopmental disorders (not all disorders are included).

Neurodevelopmental disorders in ICD-11	Neurodevelopmental disorders in DSM-5-TR
Disorders of intellectual development	Intellectual developmental disorders (intellectual disability)
Autism spectrum disorder	Autism spectrum disorder
Attention deficit hyperactivity disorder	Attention deficit/hyperactivity disorder
Developmental motor coordination disorder	Developmental coordination disorder
Developmental learning disorder	Specific learning disorder
	Tic disorders, e.g. Tourette's disorder

different features. Whereas previously conditions like autism and Asperger's were seen as more distinct, albeit very similar conditions (similar enough to create a diagnostic dilemma over whether someone had autism or Asperger's), modern terminology sees these conditions as points on a broad spectrum.

Box 1.2 **John**

John is a 25-year-old ex-solicitor. He was originally referred as an 8-year-old to see a paediatrician for possible dyspraxia before being diagnosed two years later with Asperger's syndrome. This was followed with being diagnosed with attention deficit hyperactivity disorder (ADHD) just after starting university. He recently left his job after developing a severe anxiety disorder and is currently tutoring law students online from his home in Cambridge. He has always had insomnia, but has found that not having to work 'office hours' has worsened his sleep–wake routine and he has just started taking melatonin to help with this. He is wondering if he needs to see the adult autism team to have his Asperger's diagnosis reclassified as autism.

Medical models and social models

This title of this book contains the word 'disorders', but is that the correct term for a person with a neurodevelopmental condition?

When viewed from a clinical point of view, the reasons for the word choice are clear. People do not go to an autism clinic (for example) out of a sense of curiosity. It is generally because they are experiencing difficulties of some sort and they (or their carers/parents/partners) are seeking an explanation for these difficulties and/or some kind of support. But are those difficulties necessarily down to an individual's innate make-up?

As we see in the case of Jane (Box 1.3), while there may have been notable differences in behaviour from an early age and she was subsequently diagnosed as being autistic, Jane was doing perfectly well until there was a lot of upheaval in her life (because of events not within her control), and once things were resolved she settled down again.

Is it therefore fair in Jane's case to see the autism as a disorder/disability or even as a medical condition when she is perfectly fine in the right environment? This argument can be generalised to state

Box 1.3 **Jane**

Jane is a 12-year-old who has been referred by her school with concerns about autism. She was always felt to be a little different to others in class (and at nursery), with unusual interests and a dislike for loud noises. But she was top of her class in all subjects. However, she began to experience problems after her parents separated and she went to live with her mother and new partner. Then she started a new school where she was severely bullied, including being subjected to online abuse; this led to significant school absences followed by concerns that she was developing an anxiety disorder. After delays in support, she moved back to living with her father and went back to her old school where her issues settled down. She was seen and discharged by Child and Adolescent Mental Health Services (CAMHS). When assessed by the autism team, after a lot of discussion she received a diagnosis on the basis that she fulfilled the diagnostic criteria and that a diagnosis would open up more avenues for support if there were future difficulties.

Box 1.4 **Demian**

Demian is a 12-year-old with autism, ADHD and Tourette's disorder. At school he has struggled greatly with learning because of significant difficulties with concentration, despite a number of classroom adjustments following input from an educational psychologist. Only after commencing on methylphenidate at the age of 9 did he start to make progress and within two years had almost caught up in English. For the last year he has been struggling with tics. His friends in class are very supportive, as are his parents, but he finds the repetitive twitches very unpleasant and their increasing frequency is making him feel disheartened. His paediatrician is considering trialling a medication that may help both his ADHD and his tics.

Box 1.5 **Dyslexia**

Dyslexia affects approximately 7% of the UK population. In past centuries when there was far less emphasis on reading, would this have ever caused any problems?

that in neurodivergent individuals, if the environment is right (whether through support or leaving them alone to get on with things unhindered), then although the differences remain the disorder disappears.

But how generalisable is this viewpoint? In the case of Demian (Box 1.4), the issues seem to be more down to innate/biological features than to do with the environment. To what extent can modifying a person's environment (be it sensory stimulants, people, providing aids) completely ameliorate their difficulties? Will some biological variations always be problematic? Might some features only have been seen as difficult at certain points in history (Box 1.5)?

Seeing things through a purely biological perspective is often termed a 'medical model' (of disability), whereas looking at things through a non-biological perspective is often termed a 'social model' (of disability). While different models may be exclusively favoured by different groups, there is an argument that each model may be valid in certain circumstances, but that on their own they do not provide a complete model for how we should see these conditions.

Neurodiversity

Some of the differences conferred on people with neurodevelopmental conditions also very clearly imbue them with particular strengths and skills, and there are many well-known examples of individuals with such conditions who attribute part of their success to being different. It is also possible that in past times, or in other ways of life, these conditions may have conferred other benefits on those possessing these differences, and hence to populations with such individuals.

In this sense it is possible to begin to consider whether, and to what extent, neurodivergency reflects a natural variation in how humans experience and interact with the world around them (and how this may be of benefit to the human experience). This can be termed the neurodiversity paradigm. That is not to say that certain states may not leave individuals requiring additional needs/support, but it should lead us to think carefully about how valid the concepts around 'disorders' are, and especially so when we start to address whether certain states need to be 'cured'.

The concept of neurodiversity also makes us think about the language we use to describe these states. Are they disabilities, disorders, difficulties or merely differences/diversities? It is very possible that according to time, place and person, each of these conditions could be seen as either/all.

Intended readers

The intended readership of this book is clinicians, but some of the content will also be of interest to patients, carers and members of the general public.

Most neurodivergent people see clinicians when they are seeking a diagnosis or support with associated difficulties. As such, the focus of this book skews towards the medical model. In order to be consistent with most diagnostic frameworks, medical terminology is used throughout, including most obviously in the title, *ABC of Neurodevelopmental Disorders*. This is not to neglect the importance of the social model. Clinicians must not fail to think about how a person's environment may be having detrimental impacts on them, whether this is at home, in school, or at work, and must remember that adjustments and changes can have a very significant effect on a person's well-being.

Neurodevelopmental disorders are important conditions for all clinicians to be aware of because neurodivergent people are relatively common in all populations. Those who are neurodivergent are over-represented in certain types of clinics such as community paediatrics and psychiatry, but in addition, like everyone else, they get migraines and cancer, they require operations, and they need help with having their babies delivered. But the majority of people delivering healthcare, and those who design healthcare systems, are not neurodivergent themselves, so it is important for those in the majority to think how care can be adjusted to make delivery of care equitable for everyone. This begins with being more aware of the concepts discussed in this book. Awareness of what neurodivergent people think and feel is also important, and this book does not neglect that. As well as some vignettes written by people who identify as neurodiverse, there have been other contributions to the writing, editing and reviewing of this text by neurodivergent individuals.

What follows...

This book presents an introduction to some of the most commonly encountered or familiar neurodevelopmental conditions. It also addresses common comorbid mental health conditions, because of how frequently they co-occur in those with neurodevelopmental conditions. After careful consideration, a separate chapter on foetal alcohol spectrum disorder (FASD) has been included. FASD has not yet been classified by DSM-5-TR as a neurodevelopmental condition, but it has many features in common with neurodivergent states and it may come to be classified as such in future iterations of the DSM. It is increasingly recognised as being under-diagnosed, is preventable, and as such is a good exemplar of the role of the environment in aetiology.

Hopefully, by the end of the book, you, the reader, will come away with a broad overview of neurodiversity and neurodevelopmental disorders and understand how individuals who are neurodivergent may present in the clinical sphere, how they are assessed and how they are managed. Further reading is presented at the end of each chapter so that you may explore these evolving, important and fascinating topics in greater detail.

Further reading

American Psychiatric Association (2022). *Diagnostic and Statistical Manual of Mental Disorders*, 5e. Text Revision. Washington, DC: American Psychiatric Association Publishing.

Glatt, S.J., Faraone, S.V., and Tsuang, M.T. Is schizophrenia a neurodevelopmental disorder. In: *Schizophrenia*, 4e (ed. S.J. Glatt, S.V. Faraone, and M.T. Tsuang), ch. 9. Oxford: Oxford University Press.

Shankar, R., Perera, B., and Thomas, R.H. (2020). Epilepsy, an orphan within the neurodevelopmental family. *Journal of Neurology, Neurosurgery and Psychiatry* 91: 1245–1247.

World Health Organization. International Classification of Diseases 11th Revision. https://www.who.int/standards/classifications/classification-of-diseases

CHAPTER 2

An Introduction to ADHD and Its Presentation

Munib Haroon

OVERVIEW

- Attention deficit hyperactivity disorder (ADHD) is defined by the presence of three core presenting features: inattention, hyperactivity and impulsivity.
- ADHD develops in childhood but may not be diagnosed until adolescence or later on in adulthood.
- ADHD occurs in approximately 5% of children and 3–4% of adults in the United Kingdom.
- ADHD is strongly influenced by genetics, but there are a number of environmental risk factors including in utero exposure to tobacco smoke and alcohol, low birthweight, prematurity, a history of head injury/meningitis/encephalitis and exposure to environmental lead.
- The features of ADHD can present in many ways and can change over time.
- The presentation in women and girls can be subtle, with a tendency for more internalising features to be present as opposed to externalising features.

What is ADHD?

Attention deficit hyperactivity disorder (ADHD) is a neurodevelopmental disorder defined by the presence of three main features: inattention, hyperactivity and impulsivity.

DSM-5-TR recognises three main types (Figure 2.1), a predominantly inattentive form, a predominantly hyperactive-impulsive form and a combined form. ADHD is a chronic condition (the DSM-5-TR criteria state that features should have been present for at least six months before a diagnosis can be made), with features present during childhood (before the age of 12). However, a diagnosis may be delayed for many years after the condition starts to cause difficulties with day-to-day functioning. It is in the nature of the condition, and part of the diagnostic criteria, that the condition should interfere with day-to-day

functioning in two or more settings, such as home and school/university or at an afterschool club or at work.

History

Descriptions of people with ADHD-like symptoms can be found as far back as the 1770s with Weikard's initially anonymously published text followed by Alexander Crichton's in 1798. Nevertheless, George Still's case series stands out as a landmark in the history of ADHD with its reporting of 43 children with features including inattention and overactivity (and other features that were not hallmarks of ADHD). The study noted many of the findings recognised in modern-day clinical medicine such as the apparent male : female ratio and onset during primary school years. Yet despite labelling these features as due to a 'defect of moral control' and attributing some elements to rearing, Still was prescient in proposing a hereditary component to the condition.

Over the course of the twentieth century, what we now recognise as ADHD became attributed to brain damage, minimal brain damage, or poor child rearing, before becoming recognised as a behavioural syndrome. More recent research has highlighted its genetic underpinnings as well as the contribution made by environmental risk factors.

Epidemiology

ADHD has a prevalence of approximately 5% in children in the United Kingdom. Global prevalence estimates vary widely, with ranges of 0.1–10.2% in children and adults, with a figure of 8–10% stated for the United States. The global overall prevalence is estimated to be around 5%. ADHD occurs in about 3–4% of adults in the United Kingdom.

The male : female ratio is approximately 3 : 1. This may be partly due to differences in presentation (see Box 2.1).

ADHD persists in approximately 65% of adults who were diagnosed with ADHD as children.

ABC of Neurodevelopmental Disorders, First Edition. Edited by Munib Haroon.
© 2024 John Wiley & Sons Ltd. Published 2024 by John Wiley & Sons Ltd.

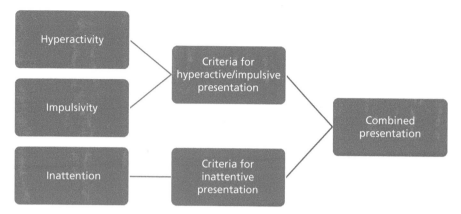

Figure 2.1 ADHD can be seen as presenting with a combined form where all three of the core features are significantly present or as a predominantly inattentive or hyperactive/impulsive presentation.

Box 2.1 **Differences in male/female presentation**

There seems to be a difference in how males and females present with ADHD. Girls and women tend to present with more internalising behaviours (inattention, anxiety, depression), while boys and men tend to present with more externalising behaviours (hyperactivity, impulsivity, conduct disorders, substance misuse). Clearly, externalised behaviour is often more apparent and does not rely on the person with the behaviour/difficulties having to understand they have a problem, communicate it to someone else and seek advice/support or help – which can be particularly problematic in childhood. Externalising behaviours can also be more disruptive in different settings and so are again more likely to lead to a referral. There may be some benefit in the use of self-report scales to help uncover internalising behaviours.

Aetiology

The genetic basis for ADHD has become increasingly clear over time. There are several strands of evidence that point to this:

- Parents of children with ADHD are between two and eight times more likely to have ADHD than parents of children without ADHD.
- Adoption studies show that adopted children tend to be more similar to their biological parents than to their adopted parents with regard to ADHD.
- Twin studies demonstrate that monozygotic twins are more similar with respect to ADHD traits than dizygotic twins.

It is now felt that genetic factors may account for more than 70–80% of the variation.

Multiple studies demonstrate that ADHD is likely to be caused in part by the interaction of many genetic variations that individually are likely to have a small effect, and may be very common, but whose overall effect is cumulative and when sufficiently aggregated in an individual can lead to the condition. There are instances, however, when a rare variant can lead to ADHD in the absence of other genetic risk factors. As well as this, studies also show the common genetic inheritance behind ADHD and conditions such as bipolar disorder and conduct disorder.

A lot of interest has focused on genes regulating dopamine and serotonin transport, because medication used to treat ADHD targets these neurotransmitters. Nevertheless, there is ongoing work to elucidate other gene variants that contribute to ADHD and the associated underlying biochemical and cellular processes and how these relate to different areas of the brain. This is being done through imaging studies, which to date have described several brain variations in those with ADHD. These include reductions in total brain volume and grey matter, delays in brain maturation, as well as variations in brain connectivity. Much of the work has focused particularly on changes to the frontal lobes and the fronto-striatal connection in people with ADHD. Slowly the links between ADHD genotype and phenotype (at the neuronal, brain and behavioural levels) are becoming clearer (see Figure 2.2).

As well as the role of genetics, it is important not to forget that non-genetic factors play an important role in the aetiology of ADHD, probably through their impact on the developing brain (see Box 2.2). These include perinatal factors such as low

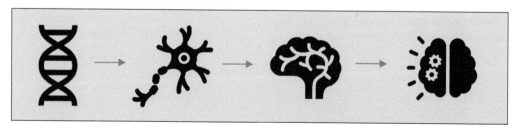

Figure 2.2 The underlying brain, neuronal and genetic basis for ADHD is becoming clearer over time.

Box 2.2 **Non-genetic risk factors for ADHD**

- Antenatal smoking
- Antenatal alcohol use
- Low birthweight
- Lead
- Traumatic brain injury
- Meningitis/encephalitis

birthweight, a history of maternal smoking and alcohol use. Environmental lead may play a role, as may traumatic brain injuries and meningitis/encephalitis.

Clinical features

The vignettes in Box 2.3 highlight some of the different ways in which ADHD can present.

Inattention

The ability to concentrate changes over time. Usually, it is a trait that improves with age. Toddlers do not focus for long periods of time on activities (and are not expected to either), and so differentiating a young child with developmentally appropriate 'inattention' from one with ADHD can be difficult. As a result, clinicians in the United Kingdom are often reluctant to make a diagnosis below the age of 6 years.

However, with age things can become clearer, and starting school can typically be a tipping point, when an inability to concentrate in a similar way to other children during lessons or other structured activities becomes clear. Children may also become aware themselves that they are unable to focus well and may report this as an issue.

Box 2.3 **Tommy and Jenna**

Tommy is 5 years old. His mum remembers him being hyperactive in utero and states that as soon as he could walk he was 'off climbing the walls'. He is accident prone and sleeps very poorly, often falling asleep after 11 p.m. and waking before 6 a.m. He finds it hard to get ready for school in the morning and has to be instructed every step of the way, from brushing his teeth to finishing his cereal to going upstairs to get changed – these often have to be repeated since he doesn't seem to take in anything as he's too busy attending to something else.

Jenna is 9 years old. She has been referred by her special educational needs coordinator (SENCO) as she is falling increasingly behind at school. She frequently forgets to do her homework or bring it in and even when she completes it, it is frequently rushed or the work does not seem to have been retained/understood. She is however a very well-behaved girl who sits at the back of class staring out of the window. She frequently returns home missing items such as books, scarves and gloves and occasionally wearing someone else's coat. She has only now been referred to see a paediatrician because she is falling more and more behind her peers and her parents have started to recognise the true extent of her difficulties.

With age, children are expected to perform increasingly difficult tasks at home and at school, and these require increasing amounts of concentration – which may lead to inattention becoming more apparent.

Inattention can present in different ways depending on age and setting and while it can be obvious, it can often 'pass under the radar' or be assumed to be something else. Sometimes there can be a different reason for apparent inattention. This can include hearing difficulties, sleep difficulties, absence seizures, anaemia, thyroid problems or learning difficulties.

While inattention needs to be pervasive for a diagnosis of ADHD to be made (it should be present in more than one setting), variations can occur. Features can sometimes be missed in a very busy or chaotic environment or in a highly structured and routinised environment – whether this is at home or at school. In addition, in free play a child with ADHD may have less noticeable features compared to their peers.

With brain maturity inattention may improve, but it tends to have the longest-lasting effects out of the three main areas of impairment. It can have a significant impact on many activities of daily living, leading to difficulties at work and home that in turn can have implications for finances and family life.

Box 2.4 demonstrates some of the ways in which the features of inattention can present on a day-to-day basis.

Hyperactivity/impulsivity

The closely related features of hyperactivity and impulsivity need to be assessed in the context of developmental age. A typical toddler might seem to have many of the symptoms discussed, but this is entirely typical for their age. At the same time, it is typical for the parents of a child with ADHD to report that their child was hyperactive from the start, sometimes as far back as in utero. Hyperactivity is also something that can become less severe with time and can occasionally recede into the background entirely or manifest as just a lot of excessive fidgeting or a feeling of restlessness. Impulsivity can remain problematic in adulthood even if the hyperactivity improves (see Box 2.5).

Box 2.6 demonstrates some of the main ways in which hyperactivity and impulsivity can present on a day-to-day basis.

Box 2.4 **Features suggestive of inattention**

- Making careless mistakes (e.g. inaccuracies when writing).
- Not remaining focused during tasks/play (e.g. switching off when reading).
- Not seeming to listen during conversations, e.g. not heeding instructions.
- Failing to complete tasks or taking a very long time to do so.
- Having organisational difficulties (e.g. being messy/disorganised, not doing a series of sequential tasks properly).
- Avoiding difficult tasks (not doing homework, procrastinating, starting things but failing to finish them).
- Losing items (reports, clothes, bags, phones).
- Being easily distracted by people, sounds and sights, and thoughts.
- Forgetting daily activities (doing chores, keeping appointments, making calls).

Box 2.5 **On ADHD**

'When I look back, I realise that I had many of the core features of ADHD. The most difficult aspect was the inattention. At school I would daydream as the teacher was speaking at the blackboard and then have to look around at what the child next to me was doing in order to understand what our task was, or how to do it, and even then I would lapse into my thoughts, only rousing myself when the lesson ended. I fell behind a lot as a result in primary school. Even whilst walking home with my grandfather, I would be aware that he was talking to me but remain lost in my thoughts until he would ask me something, and I would be oblivious to what he was referring to. "Careless boy! Careless boy!" he would chide me. Over time my features began to improve and as a result so did my schoolwork. Despite being inattentive I have always been able to hyperfocus on things that interest me. I was a little professor and once I could focus better, I was able to excel in some areas of work.'

Box 2.6 **Features suggestive of hyperactivity and impulsivity**

Hyperactivity
- Fidgeting (tapping, squirming, shuffling).
- Inability to sit still (e.g. leaving the classroom seat frequently, or leaving a desk at work).
- Excess activity (e.g. running/climbing) or feelings of restlessness.
- Inability to do activities quietly.
- Being continually on the go or feeling the need to be, e.g. inner restlessness.
- Excessive speech.

Impulsivity
- Blurting out answers or completing sentences for other people or being unable to wait for one's turn in a conversation.
- Difficulty waiting one's turn (e.g. when lining up at school, or in other queues).
- Interrupting/intruding on others.
- Inability to curb actions, e.g. running into the road or hitting people.

Other presenting features

People with ADHD also have difficulties with emotional regulation and may experience issues such as anger, impatience, frustration and hostility. This may be linked to and overlap with conditions such as oppositional defiant disorder and conduct disorder. There is also an association with low self-esteem, which can, over time, tip over into depression. People with ADHD typically report feeling on edge and restless; when excessive this can be one of the pointers that there is a coexistent anxiety disorder.

Clearly, these features can have wide impacts on day-to-day functioning and affect relationships, but also learning and work. As has been stressed, it is quite usual for neurodevelopmental conditions not to exist in isolation, and so it is common for people with ADHD to present with tics or have features attributable to autism. Sometimes these other conditions may be more apparent and make it harder for the ADHD to be recognised.

Conclusion

ADHD is a chronic neurodevelopmental condition that usually manifests in childhood, but can continue to cause difficulties long into adulthood because of its core and related features. As such, it can intrude into most aspects of daily life, including family life, education, work and leisure activities. There are thus compelling reasons to diagnose the condition and address its management at an early stage.

Further reading

American Psychiatric Association (2022). *Diagnostic and Statistical Manual of Mental Disorders*, 5e. Text Revision. Washington, DC: American Psychiatric Association Pusblishing.

Barkley, R.A. (2018). *Attention-Deficit Hyperactivity Disorder*, 4e. New York: Guilford Press.

Faraone, S.V. and Larsson, H. (2019). Genetics of attention deficit hyperactivity disorder. *Molecular Psychiatry* 24: 562–575.

Selikowitz, M. (2021). *ADHD: The Facts*. Oxford: Oxford University Press.

Stibbe, T., Huang, J., Paucke, M. et al. (2020). Gender differences in adult ADHD: cognitive function assessed by the test of attentional performance. *PLoS One* 15 (10): e0240810. https://doi.org/10.1371/journal.pone.0240810.

CHAPTER 3

The Assessment and Diagnosis of ADHD in Children and Young People

Ayesha Qureshi

OVERVIEW

- The diagnosis of ADHD is dependent on obtaining a clear history and conducting a thorough examination.
- Obtaining information on the symptoms/signs/presentation in more than one setting/domain is crucial.
- It is important not to neglect the voice of the child.
- Assessment should include the voice/thoughts/impressions of the child.
- There is no role for routine biomedical tests.
- Diagnosis requires assessment against the DSM/ICD criteria following a full clinical and psychosocial assessment.

Referrals for suspected ADHD

In the United Kingdom, assessment and diagnosis are carried out by specialists working in secondary care (community paediatricians or child and adolescent psychiatrists). Referrals come to secondary care from various professionals including school/educational psychology, social care and other doctors/healthcare professionals. Often school referrals come from the special educational needs coordinator (SENCO). Sometimes the GP may act as a conduit for these, but not always (see Figure 3.1).

Before referral to secondary care, enquiries should be made about how pervasive the difficulties are. A GP may suggest a watchful waiting period of 10 weeks prior to referral and want to obtain a report from the school.

Important points for the referrer to consider include: How long have concerns been present? What are the specific difficulties and how do they affect the child's family and school life? Have any strategies been put in place, such as parenting/school behavioural support? How did these strategies affect the child's presentation?

Integrated working can be very useful during the referral process, with simultaneous referral of the family to any local parent programmes or family support. How this is presented to parents can be key to their engagement. For example, telling a parent 'We are referring you to parenting classes' can make them feel judged negatively and disempowered. The aim should be to open a discussion with the family about avenues of more specific support (ADHD parent training classes) and how these may provide useful information and strategies to manage stressful situations. Hearing carers' difficulties empathetically is important for their future interactions with services. Empowering them is important for the benefit of their child.

Setting realistic expectations early in the process can be helpful for all involved. Specialist centres will not assess before the age of 5 or 6 years, as it is important to differentiate a normal from an abnormal level of activity, taking a child's developmental stage into account.

Some families may be living in adverse circumstances or dealing with challenging social conditions – this can have a significant impact on presentation. The effect of the difficulties can be enhanced if, for instance, they are living in overcrowded conditions, with no access to a safe outside space for play, or dealing with stretched parenting capacity, such as where there are multiple young children with no support for the parent. Such set-ups may prompt an earlier interaction with primary care, requesting a referral for assessment.

Recently more parents are being assessed and diagnosed with ADHD themselves. They may see similarities in their child, and this may be another reason they approach primary care for a referral for their child.

Referrals are typically triaged by a specialist service to ensure that the appropriate criteria have been met. It is important to include as much relevant information as possible in the initial referral. Most services have referral forms, which may guide the referrer to the information required. Good referrals help reduce any bounce-back that may occur otherwise. In addition, emotional/behavioural difficulty referrals without evidence of ADHD warrant consideration for different routes of support, for instance local family support agencies, and not to a specialist ADHD clinic. At times there may be redirection to alternative services if it is not thought that ADHD assessment is the current correct route.

ABC of Neurodevelopmental Disorders, First Edition. Edited by Munib Haroon.
© 2024 John Wiley & Sons Ltd. Published 2024 by John Wiley & Sons Ltd.

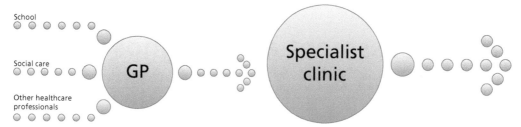

Figure 3.1 The route to a specialist clinic often involves the GP, either directly, or with them acting as a conduit. Referral may come from schools/social care or other healthcare professionals.

What happens at the specialist clinic?

Centres will have varying team set-ups. The team could include ADHD specialist nurses, psychologists, paediatricians and psychiatrists. In some centres the team may be more medically led.

Collation of information from more than one domain (e.g. from school *and* parents) remains essential to any assessment process for ADHD. Once someone is accepted into the service, the common theme is acquiring a full clinical history and conducting a wider psychosocial assessment. This includes investigating behaviours and symptoms in the different domains and settings of the person's everyday life and conducting a full developmental history.

Screening questionnaires may be requested with the referral or after the first assessment. These need to be done across two domains, the second generally being an education setting. There are various versions available such as Conners and Vanderbilt screening questionnaires. A Strengths and Difficulties Questionnaire (SDQ) may also be requested.

Some clinics may have access to psychometric testing or a Quantitative Behavioural Test (QbTest). This is a computer-based test delivered directly to the patient that measures core ADHD symptoms. The test results are analysed and presented in a report that compares a patient's results with a group of people of the same age and sex who do not have ADHD.

History

A conducive environment is essential to obtaining a history from the parents or carers with all the relevant details. The attendance of a teacher or SENCO who knows the child well, if the parents agree, can also be very useful. The history helps build a picture of whether the difficulties are in keeping with ADHD or otherwise. Sometimes ADHD may co-occur with other conditions. With neurodevelopmental conditions there can be a great deal of overlap, but defining a primary difficulty can be helpful. However, it is also not straightforward. For instance, with a child on the autistic spectrum, whether the excess movement is related to sensory processing differences rather than inherent hyperactivity may require some unpicking.

A psychosocial/developmental history is essential. Traumatic events/adverse childhood experiences are important aspects of the history. This may be particularly relevant in families where there have already been child safeguarding interventions or indeed for children who are in local authority care. Neurodevelopmental trauma can present with the symptoms of ADHD. There can be

significant levels of anxiety or oppositional features in such presentations. Such a history does not automatically exclude an ADHD diagnosis; however, the information holds important prognostic value. It will inform the clinician and aid them with realistic counselling related to diagnosis and management, because treatment can be less efficacious.

A number of aspects of the past medical history and family history should be enquired about. This includes the presence of any first-degree relatives with congenital or childhood acquired heart conditions or with a history of arrhythmias as well as the presence of any sudden unexpected death in childhood (SUDIC). If such a history is present in a child who is subsequently diagnosed with ADHD, an electrocardiogram (ECG) should be carried out prior to commencing a child on medication.

It is important not to focus solely on what is said by parents/carers. Where a child is old enough, their perspective should be part of the assessment. Often comments from even young children can be highly revealing. Sometimes they may give very insightful descriptions:

- 'My brain goes too fast, and I can't get it on to the paper.'
- 'It's all jumbled up in my head and it's like switching between computer screens too fast.'
- 'The teacher tells me something and I think I get it but then I still can't do it and I don't know why.'
- 'Sometimes I only get the first bit and get stuck, but then I don't want to ask and look stupid.'

It may be useful to ask the parents/carers to forward on any relevant additional written information that is felt to be too sensitive to discuss there and then. This can help to minimise the child/young person feeling criticised or being diminished to a list of negative behaviours.

Examination

As well as conducting a physical observation, it is important to spend time observing the child/young person – and this may start from the moment they are greeted in the waiting room. Observation of how the child interacts with their space, the examiner and their parents is important information.

Any pre-existing diagnoses, such as autism, should be taken into account, with appropriate adjustments made where necessary. For instance, there may be significant social anxiety or difficulties with communication to be considered.

Box 3.1 **Features to note on the examination of a child with possible ADHD**

- General assessment and growth and nutrition parameters
- Developmental attainment
- Attention, impulsivity and hyperactivity
- Presence of comorbid conditions and other differentials, including previous head trauma
- Neurocutaneous stigmata
- Skin stigmata of neurofibromatosis or tuberous sclerosis (using a Wood's light)
- Signs of injury or multiple bruises in non-worrying areas (may indicate a high level of activity)
- Signs of maltreatment/neglect/abuse
- Features of foetal alcohol spectrum disorder
- Signs of self-harm
- Congenital anomalies and dysmorphic features, including micro/macrocephaly
- Neurological signs
- Cardiovascular examination (the presence of any abnormalities)
- Tics
- Genetic conditions such as Prader-Willi/Fragile X/DiGeorge

Box 3.2 **Differential diagnosis and comorbid conditions when assessing a child for possible ADHD**

Neurodevelopment, mental health or behavioural disorders
- Autism
- Intellectual disability
- Global developmental delay
- Traumatic brain injury
- Developmental coordination disorder
- Conduct disorder
- Oppositional defiant disorder
- Psychosis
- Mood disorder
- Anxiety disorder
- Attachment disorders
- Obsessive compulsive disorder
- Foetal alcohol spectrum disorder
- Genetic disorders, e.g. Klinefelter/Marfan/Fragile X/Prader-Willi
- Substance misuse

Other conditions
- Hearing impairment
- Severe visual impairment
- Maltreatment

Some children cannot sit still: they will climb, run and touch every item they can in the room. They may show fleeting attention to toys; older children may clearly zone out and be unable to concentrate at all. Alternatively, the parents may comment that the child is unusually well behaved and not showing their true colours. The ability to sit still and focus for a short period of time, in a novel (and potentially interesting) setting, should not be used on its own to rule out a diagnosis of ADHD.

Where children have florid hyperactivity/impulsivity and are jumping around the room, interrupting frequently and displaying poor impulse control, it is important to put safety first while trying to be adaptable and flexible.

A full physical examination should occur, keeping in mind the features in Box 3.1.

Sometimes a full examination cannot be completed in one session. The initial assessment may also highlight the need to consider onward referrals, for instance to the geneticist/cardiologist/endocrinologist. There are a number of differential diagnoses and comorbid conditions that a clinician should be aware of and that may prompt further assessments/referrals (see Box 3.2).

Biomedical tests

Medical investigations should not be routinely carried out but should be considered on an individual basis. An ECG may be required if there is a history of cardiac anomalies in first-degree relatives or SUDIC. Other tests may be required depending on the presence of dysmorphology, neurocutaneous lesions, congenital abnormalities or intellectual disability.

The clinical history may prompt some other tests. For example, if there are concerns about a child daydreaming/zoning out frequently and not being attentive when called back to attention, a hyperventilation test in clinic and an electroencephalogram (EEG)

may be needed to exclude absence seizures. Audiology assessments should be considered to exclude a hearing impairment causing inattention.

Diagnosis

A diagnosis of ADHD should only be made by a specialist psychiatrist, paediatrician or other appropriately qualified healthcare professional with training and expertise in the diagnosis of ADHD. This will be based on a full clinical and psychosocial assessment of the person. This should include discussion about behaviour and symptoms across the different domains and settings of their everyday life and a full developmental and psychiatric history and observer reports (e.g. as gathered from before the clinical assessment) and assessment of the person's mental state along with a full physical exam (see Figure 3.2).

The diagnosis should not be made solely based on a rating scale or observational data. However, rating scales such as the Conners rating scales and the SDQ are valuable adjuncts, and observations

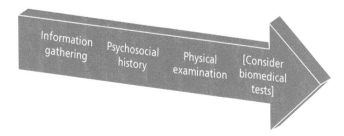

Figure 3.2 The assessment and diagnosis of ADHD consist of several steps, beginning with preliminary information gathering prior to a clinic assessment.

(for example at school) are useful when there is doubt about symptoms. The assessment should lead to consideration around whether a child has ADHD (symptoms of hyperactivity/impulsivity and/or inattention) based on the current DSM-5-TR (or ICD-11) criterion. Salient features to consider are:

- The presence of several features suggestive of the inattentive form, the hyperactive/impulsive form or the combined form, which must have been present from before the age of 12.
- Features should cause at least moderate psychological, social and/or educational or occupational impairment based on interview and/or direct observation. They should be pervasive, occurring in two or more important settings, such as at home, school, work or other social setting.
- The diagnostic process should include an assessment of the child's needs, coexisting conditions, social, familial and educational context and physical health. There should also be some assessment of their parents' or carers' mental health.
- ADHD should be considered in all age groups, with symptom criteria adjusted for age-appropriate changes in behaviour.
- Children and young people's views should be considered wherever possible in determining the clinical significance of impairment resulting from the symptoms of ADHD.

Diagnostic counselling

Diagnostic counselling is a very important part of the child's journey and will require an overview of all the processes already discussed. The diagnosis should be fed back sensitively and informatively to the carers/parents/family and to the child themselves (wherever possible) in a collaborative way.

It is imperative to discuss what the condition entails and any comorbidities. This helps prevent any misunderstanding about the diagnosis and indeed the realistic outcomes of any management or treatment measures. A full report is prepared after the assessment process. The diagnosis is shared with the family and their GP and any educational establishment (with consent). In the case of non-diagnosis, the outcome needs to be discussed openly and information shared as appropriate. The family should be directed to appropriate resources for further information.

Further reading

National Institute for Health and Care Excellence (2018). Attention deficit hyperactivity disorder: diagnosis and management. NICE guideline [NG87]. www.nice.org.uk/guidance/ng87/resources/attention-deficit-hyperactivity-disorder-diagnosis-and-management-pdf-1837699732933

CHAPTER 4

The Treatment and Outcomes of Children and Young People with ADHD

Munib Haroon

OVERVIEW

- Maintaining a good lifestyle with appropriate sleep hygiene, good nutrition and exercise is important in the management of ADHD.
- Environmental modifications along with behavioural interventions and programmes are an important part of managing ADHD.
- Medication is important where symptoms are causing persistent and significant impairment in at least one domain after environmental modifications have been implemented and reviewed.
- Medication should be commenced after appropriate assessment and discussion with the child/young person and caregivers.
- Medication should be given in line with the British National Formulary (in the UK) and appropriate guidelines.

The management of ADHD depends on several factors, including the age of the child/young person, the severity of the condition, and the presence of comorbid or other underlying conditions. Good advice, though free, is not always easy to come by, but everyone should be offered advice and support around what the condition is and how it can affect the individual and their families, and be provided with guidance around positive approaches to interactions, consistent approaches to behaviour and the value of structured routines.

Advice on optimising good sleep patterns, obtaining plenty of exercise (see Box 4.1) and good nutrition should not be neglected, and ignoring these factors may lead to suboptimal outcomes with other treatment modalities. Everyone with ADHD should have access to some sort of behavioural intervention, whether this is a parent training programme or other behaviour-based training, which may be group based. Cognitive behavioural therapy (CBT) can be useful as an adjunct to medication to help with social skills, problem solving, self-control, active listening and dealing with feelings.

Environmental modifications are important considerations. At home this may be modifications to help with sleep (like reducing extraneous noise, using blackout curtains, or limiting time on tablets and other electronic devices) or other measures that are generic and similar to those used at school (albeit adapted to a home environment).

In school these adjustments/adaptations can take a number of forms and are shown in Box 4.2. Reducing sensory overload could involve looking at lighting in the classroom or the amount of distracting material on tables and walls, or the use of earphones. Appropriate seating may involve having the child sitting close to the teacher, further away from distracting peers, and/or them having the opportunity to spend time at a desk on their own. Aids such as timers and visual timetables or diaries can be helpful. It is important to think about how pupils with ADHD are given instructions in term of length, complexity and whether auditory instructions may be supplemented with written ones. Time away from class can be helpful, as can the use of teaching assistants and more one-to-one time.

There are different approaches to how schools will achieve these adaptations. In principle this involves making a determination that support is required, putting a modification in place, measuring the outcome and deciding if the instigated measure is sufficient or not, then repeating the cycle as required in a timely fashion.

Medication

Medication for ADHD is not licensed in the United Kingdom for children under the age of 6 years. When used, it tends to be for ADHD at the moderate to severe end of severity, where symptoms are causing persistent and significant issues in at least one area of life (such as at home or at school) after adjustments have been put in place to try to help. In the United Kingdom, medication is initiated and supervised by a specialist – usually a community paediatrician or a psychiatrist – with shared-care arrangements in place with primary care organisations allowing for monitoring and ongoing prescribing of medication.

Medications used for managing ADHD may be stimulants such as methylphenidate (see Figure 4.1). All have a side-effect profile that prescribers and 'users' should be aware of. As such, the decision to prescribe is made on a pros and cons basis following a discussion between clinician, patient and caregiver (where appropriate) and should take information from school/college into account. Parents and caregivers should have ample opportunity to think about the options, and medication information leaflets can serve as useful

---

ABC of Neurodevelopmental Disorders, First Edition. Edited by Munib Haroon.
© 2024 John Wiley & Sons Ltd. Published 2024 by John Wiley & Sons Ltd.

Box 4.1 **M, ADHD and exercise**

'When I started running at university it was transformative. Suddenly I was able to focus as I had never been able to before. The effect didn't last forever, perhaps for half the day (sometimes more) but this was significant. I also lost a lot of weight and felt healthier, and this helped my self-esteem. I slept better, and the constant gnawing edge of anxiety that always seemed to prey on my mind was suddenly banished on the days when I laced up my trainers.'

Box 4.2 **Adjustments/adaptations that schools can consider to help a student with ADHD**

- Reducing sensory overload/distractions
- Seating, e.g. pupil placement relative to teacher, wobble cushions
- Peer placement (who they sit next to)
- Timers
- Visual timetables
- Appropriate instruction length/complexity
- Timeout cards/opportunities
- Teaching assistants or more one-to-one time

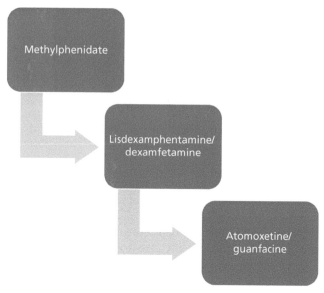

Figure 4.1 Different medications should be used in a step-wise progression according to appropriate national guidance (in the United Kingdom this is guidance from NICE).

adjuncts to this. It is also important to assess the patient for the presence of possible contraindications and to think about the need for further investigations. The National Institute for Health and Care Excellence (NICE) guideline lists when referral to a cardiologist should take place prior to commencing medication (see Box 4.3).

Baseline monitoring should also be done prior to medicating. This should include a review of mental health, thinking about the presence of/impact on other neurodevelopmental conditions, and also address educational or employment issues and safeguarding issues. Physical health measures should be taken with a focus on the

Box 4.3 **NICE guidance on referral to a cardiologist for further cardiac tests prior to commencing medication**

Referral to a cardiologist should be made when one of the following exists:
- History of congenital heart disease or cardiac surgery.
- Sudden death in first-degree relative aged <40 years where cardiac disease was felt to be an issue.
- Dyspnoea on exertion more notable relative to peers.
- Fainting on exertion or to fright/noise.
- Palpitations that are rapid, regular and start and stop suddenly.
- Chest pain that could be cardiac.
- A heart murmur.
- Signs of heart failure.

Raised blood pressure that is consistently above the 95th centile for age and height should prompt referral to a hypertension specialist.

Box 4.4 **NICE guidance on monitoring the effects of medication**

- Height: six-monthly.
- Weight: three-monthly in those aged 10 years and under.
- Weight: three and six months after starting medication and then six-monthly if over 10 years.
- Blood pressure and pulse: after every dose change and then six-monthly.
- Medication review: at least yearly.
- Specialist/trained professional review for compliance, symptoms of ADHD, adverse effects, benefit of medication.

presence of possible contraindications and include height, weight and blood pressure (and also a cardiovascular examination in general).

Medication should be started at a low dose and slowly titrated to obtain the right balance between symptoms control and minimisation of side effects. This requires appropriate and ongoing monitoring (see Box 4.4). A written treatment plan can be helpful for parents/carers and teachers alike.

In the majority of patients, the first medication to be trialled will be a form of methylphenidate. The decision to switch to an alternative often occurs when the medication does not seem to be controlling symptoms adequately (for example after having commenced it and trialled it for six weeks) or where the side effects are deemed intolerable. Alternatively, a second-line medication may be used because a medication is contraindicated.

Occasionally two different medications may be used in an effort to reduce the side effects of a medication that is otherwise working well, but where additional symptom control is required.

Methylphenidate

A stimulant and controlled medication; this is generally the first line of treatment. Methylphenidate comes in short-acting or prolonged-release forms. Increasingly the prolonged-release form is used from the start as it is more convenient; however, the short-acting form can serve as a useful adjunct.

Medication is usually given first thing in the morning, although additional doses may be required around lunchtime, after school or in the early evening.

Stimulants are associated with several side effects, ranging from common to rare and from mild to severe; however, the medication is generally well tolerated. Among the commonest effects reported are increased mood lability, which often settles down in about a week, but blood pressure and pulse (typically raised a mild amount) and appetite suppression (and hence growth) need ongoing monitoring. Stimulants, especially the longer-lasting ones, can interfere with sleep, although in a patient with significant hyperactivity they can be helpful in achieving a calmer environment. Patients with other neurodevelopmental conditions can be especially sensitive to their effects.

It is important to note that while the Children's British National Formulary (BNF) gives guidance for prescribing for children between the ages of 4 and 6 years, methylphenidate is not licensed for use in children under the age of 6 in the United Kingdom.

Lisdexamphetamine

This medication is another central nervous system stimulant and is a controlled drug, often used as a second-line medication. It has a similar side-effect profile to methylphenidate, but seems to be provide better round-the-clock effects in some patients.

Atomoxetine

A non-stimulant, selective noradrenaline reuptake inhibitor (SNRI), atomoxetine is generally used if the previous two agents have not worked. It was often considered useful in children who also had tics, but while it does not exacerbate them, it is not particularly helpful in treating them either. It does tend to cause less appetite suppression than methylphenidate. Although the side-effect profile is similar to methylphenidate, it is not identical, and two potential risks that patients and carers should be aware of and know the signs to look out for (despite their being rare) are suicidality and the risk of liver impairment and failure.

Guanfacine

This can be useful where other agents have not led to an acceptable reduction of symptoms or where the side effects were unacceptable. It is particularly useful when faced with a situation where medications are leading to appetite suppression and also where a patient has coexisting tics, as guanfacine has been shown to effectively treat tics.

Alternative Agents

These can include clonidine and atypical antipsychotics, but NICE advises obtaining a second opinion or referral to a tertiary service.

Outcomes

There is increasing recognition that ADHD can persist well into adulthood, with 65% of those diagnosed with ADHD continuing to have symptoms as adults (including those in partial remission). The evidence is that children who are treated may experience better outcomes than those who are not treated, although these outcomes are not identical to those of healthy individuals who do not have ADHD.

Further reading

Arnold, L.E., Hodgkins, P., Kahle, K. et al. (2020). Long term outcomes of ADHD: academic achievement and performance. *Journal of Attention Disorders* 24 (1): 73–85.

Barkley, R.A. (2015). *Attention-Deficit Hyperactivity Disorder*, 4e. New York: Guilford Press.

Keilow, M., Holm, A., and Fallesen, P. Medical treatment of attention deficit/hyperactivity disorder (ADHD) and children's academic performance. *PLoS One* 13 (11): e0207905. doi: 10.1371/journal.pone.0207905.

National Institute for Health and Care Excellence (2018). Attention deficit hyperactivity disorder: diagnosis and management. NICE guideline [NG87]. www.nice.org.uk/guidance/ng87/resources/attention-deficit-hyperactivity-disorder-diagnosis-and-management-pdf-1837699732933

Shaw, M., Hodgkins, P., Caci, H. et al. (2012). A systematic review and analysis of long-term outcomes in attention deficit hyperactivity disorder: effects of treatment and non-treatment. *BMC Medicine* 10: 99.

CHAPTER 5

ADHD: Adult Considerations

Munib Haroon

OVERVIEW

- ADHD is a developmental disorder that can often persist into adulthood but may not be diagnosed until post 18.

- The assessment of ADHD in adults should be holistic and include a full clinical and psychosocial, developmental history, and observer reports.

- A diagnosis should be made when a person fulfils the ICD-11 or DSM-5-TR criteria.

- ADHD in adulthood is associated with a number of areas of difficulty and poorer outcomes. These include outcomes in education, employment, social functioning and mental and physical health.

- Studies show increased all-cause mortality in adults with ADHD and notably increased rates attributable to unnatural causes such as suicide and unintentional injuries.

Key features

ADHD in adults may be seen in the context of a diagnosis made in childhood, but while the condition or its symptoms can often persist into adulthood, sometimes the features may only come to cause concern or become associated with a possible diagnosis of ADHD after the age of 18.

Transitional care, assessment and making a diagnosis in adulthood

Transitioning into adulthood

One possible situation is where a young adult with known ADHD is no longer felt to need medication (or has decided that they do not need it), but the core and associated features continue to persist. Without the requirement for being followed up for medication, there may be very little medical or formal input (other than patient support groups) and such people with ADHD may feel as if they have to 'muddle through' life unsatisfactorily.

Where young adults require ongoing supervision into adulthood, because they continue to need ADHD medication, it is crucial that there are adequate transitional care arrangements in place so that their journey from a paediatric to an adult patient can be as uncomplicated as possible. This requires early planning and discussion between all relevant parties and good documentation.

ADHD features in adulthood

In adulthood, inattention, impulsivity and a degree of restlessness often continue to characterise the condition. This can lead to difficulties in a number of areas, such as completing tasks, procrastinating over whether to start tasks, losing track of reading, impatience, difficulty relaxing, organisational problems, verbal impulsivity, making rash decisions and a poor memory (see Box 5.1). In addition, the poor self-esteem seen in many children with ADHD can continue into adulthood, as can issues to do with mood and anxiety. Mental health issues are commonly seen. Similarly, the impact of difficulties with learning in childhood can mount up, leading to poor learning outcomes as an adult. The need for stimulation can lead to adults taking part in high-risk activities, some of which can be addictive, such as substance use (which is sometimes seen as a type of self-medication) and gambling. Different aspects of the condition can therefore have an impact on relationships, ongoing education, employment and day-to-day life.

Having ADHD does not stop a person from driving, but if the symptoms or medication have an impact on driving, then in the United Kingdom the Driver and Vehicle Licensing Agency (DVLA) needs to be informed.

Assessment in adults

An increasingly common presentation occurs when a previously undiagnosed adult seeks an assessment for ADHD. In this situation the principles of assessment are similar to the assessment of a child. There is no diagnostic test, and diagnosis is reliant on a detailed history and clinical examination with the use of psychometric testing.

Because ADHD is, by definition, a neurodevelopmental disorder, there is a presumption that in order to be diagnosed, a person must have had impairments or deficits in the areas affected by ADHD during childhood – specifically before the age of 12 – and that their issues are not better explained by another (psychiatric) condition, plus the symptoms are causing moderate/severe psychological, social, educational or occupational harm. But once a person has left school, childhood issues might be difficult to demonstrate unless they have kept school reports, and it becomes increasingly difficult to do this if there is no ready access to a parent or someone else who remembers them from childhood. Although what a person can recall about themselves is also important.

The assessment also entails ruling out differentials and considering comorbidities. This includes conditions encountered in childhood, such as autism, but also conditions that are rare in children, such as bipolar disorder, the schizophrenia spectrum and psychotic and personality disorders.

As with children, it is important to be aware that ADHD has an increased prevalence in particular groups and that it is under-recognised in females and in those from certain ethnic groups.

The assessment should be holistic and include a full clinical, psychosocial and developmental history, and also observer reports. A diagnosis should be made when a person fulfils the ICD-11 or DSM-5-TR criteria.

Treatment

Following a new diagnosis, the affected adult should have a structured discussion about the implications of a diagnosis. A treatment plan as well as communication with relevant professionals, such as other healthcare providers and educational establishments, can be helpful. Good lifestyle practices should be encouraged (diet, sleep, exercise, limiting substance use) and environmental changes in the home/workplace/university addressed.

Medication

Medication is offered to adults when they have significant and ongoing issues in at least one area of life (such as home or work) after environmental modifications have been implemented and reviewed. Where medication alone is sub-optimal, a non-pharmacological therapy can be added such as psychological interventions or cognitive behavioural therapy (CBT). Non-pharmacological interventions may be the best option for those who do not want medication, where adherence is not possible or where it is ineffective or not tolerated.

In adults, lisdexamphentamine or methylphenidate is the first-line pharmacological treatment (lisdexamphetamine is off label for adults without symptoms in childhood). Atomoxetine is recommended where lisdexamphetamine or methylphenidate are not tolerated or are ineffective after a six-week trial. Medications such as guanfacine or antipsychotics should only be considered after a second opinion or following assessment by a tertiary service (see Figure 5.1).

The impact of medication can be significant (see Box 5.2).

Maintenance and monitoring of medication

Weight and blood pressure should be checked every six months and patients assessed for dose effectiveness and adverse effects. As with children, it is important to monitor adherence and be aware of the risk of stimulant diversion. Medication may need to be long term, but that should not be an automatic presumption and, as well as considering whether a particular medication and the dose are optimal, thought should be given to stopping medication periodically as a trial or reducing the dose.

Prognosis

ADHD in adulthood is associated with a number of areas of difficulty and poorer outcomes. These include outcomes in education, employment and social functioning; there is also a higher incidence of mental and physical health issues such as illicit substance use and obesity. The core features of ADHD itself may contribute to these outcomes, as may associated features and the presence of comorbidities.

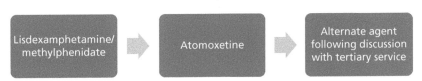

Figure 5.1 Medication for ADHD should be prescribed sequentially according to NICE guidance.

Box 5.2 **R on having ADHD**

'For years, I knew that my brain worked differently – I was what many call "neurodivergent". I had occasional bouts of anxiety, intrusive thoughts, and also an inability to concentrate or focus on certain activities, work or tasks. The words "doesn't concentrate" were all over my school reports growing up. For anything to get my attention and focus, it either required genuinely critical deadlines (and I would make sure I hit the deadline, but by doing the work at the very last possible moment), or that it was a topic that I found genuinely and personally interesting.

Once I graduated, while my symptoms were there, they didn't appear to get in the way of my life too much, as I had developed a good awareness of how I thought and operated, and so I developed my own coping mechanisms. However, there were two things that I was unable to manage; the first were the migraines that I had from an early age, and the second was the constant tiredness and fatigue. I tried many things to find the source of this fatigue and the migraines. I had tests, looked at my lifestyle, but nothing seemed to solve it. I eventually blamed the tiredness on my hectic life with young kids and long work hours.

About a year ago, I decided it was time to dig deeper into my mental health. My symptoms were the same, but I wanted to understand why I was the way I was. I needed to know what was going on in my head.

I met with a psychiatrist who, after hours of discussion and using a tool called the DIVA assessment, concluded that I had ADHD. I wasn't entirely convinced at first, but over the hours we spent together, I started to agree more and more with him, until I felt almost entirely confident in his diagnosis. It explained a lot!

I hadn't considered medication when I first reached out to the psychiatrist, so the idea took me by surprise. But, after some thought, I decided to try it out.

What has been the impact of the medicine on my life? It's like this: you know that feeling of grogginess when you immediately wake up in the morning? Well, that's how I felt. ALL THE TIME. Now, with the medication, I feel… Awake. Aware. Attentive. I'm here. It has been transformational. And incidentally, after several months, I've also had fewer migraines which I think is down to better sleep. Going through it all has been life-changing.'

There are limited studies addressing life expectancy in those with ADHD, but studies show an increased all-cause mortality and notably increased rates attributable to unnatural causes such as suicide and unintentional injuries (Table 5.1). While the presence of other comorbid/psychiatric conditions may augment this risk, ADHD itself seems to be a significant risk factor.

Qualitative evidence and evidence from individual studies have suggested that treatment may reduce many of these risks. One meta-analysis (addressing studies across all age ranges) demonstrated that medication (predominantly with stimulants) could achieve statistically significant improvements with respect to accidents and injuries and improvements in mood disorders. There were also improved outcomes for criminality, substance use disorders, suicidality and traumatic brain injury, albeit these did not achieve statistical significance. The effects on academic outcomes was more mixed, although studies overall tended to support improved outcomes with medication.

Criminal justice system

The vast majority of individuals with ADHD do not commit criminal offences. But there is an association between ADHD and becoming involved in criminal behaviour and doing so at an earlier age compared to individuals without ADHD. A number of studies show that the prevalence of ADHD among the incarcerated population is at least 20%. This may, in part, be due to the core issue of impulsivity, which may lead to individuals with ADHD acting without thinking about the consequences of their actions. Those with ADHD also show more risk-taking behaviours. When the ADHD is coupled with oppositional defiant disorder or conduct disorder (CD) or other comorbid diagnoses (for example substance abuse), the risk increases further and there is evidence that comorbid CD and ADHD are better predictors of criminality than ADHD alone.

The heritable aspects of ADHD may also partly contribute to experiencing adverse life events, traumatic circumstances and abuse in childhood, which can then have long-term effects on behaviour. Inattention can lead to poor academic performance, which may reduce job prospects and may be an additional factor.

Conclusion

The features of ADHD can cast a long shadow over those affected by it, but identification and appropriate treatment of ADHD are associated with improved outcomes. As has hopefully been shown in this chapter, the prospects do not need to be bleak despite the statistics, and people with ADHD can lead highly productive lives even in the face of persisting features.

Table 5.1 ADHD is associated with an increased overall risk of death in adults with the condition, as well as an increased risk of death due to 'unnatural' causes, compared to those without ADHD.

Study and type	Participant details	Outcomes
Schiavone et al. (2022) Prospective perinatal risk cohort study	1196 infants with predefined perinatal risks Follow up of n = 839 at 46 years of those with: • Childhood ADHD (n = 115) • Attentional problems (n = 216) • No attentional problems (n = 508)	All-cause mortality ADHD (compared to no/low ADHD) Adjusted hazard ratio [95% CI] (p): 2.15 [1.02, 4.54] (0.04) Mortality before 30 years: 6.2 [1.78, 21.57] (0.004) Mortality for unnatural causes of death: 2.82 [1.12, 7.12] (0.03)
Dalsgaard et al. (2015) Danish nationwide cohort study	1.9 million individuals followed up (32 061 with ADHD) 5580 cohort member deaths (107 with ADHD)	ADHD MRR adjusted [95% CI] (p) 2.07 [1.7–2.5] (<0.0001) Age at first diagnosis vs MRR 1–5 yr = 1.86 [0.93, 3.27] 6–17 yr = 1.58 [1.21–2.03] >17 yr = 4.25 (3.03–5.78) No ADHD = 1.00 ADHD + ODD/CD + SUD = 8.74 [5.12–13.80] 79/107 deaths in ADHD individuals were identified 54/79 deaths were due to 'unnatural causes'
Sun et al. (2019) Swedish nationwide cohort study	2.6 million individuals (86 670 with ADHD) 6655 cohort member deaths (424 with ADHD)	ADHD (relative to controls) Adjusted HR [95% CI] All-cause mortality: 3.94 [3.51–4.43] Adulthood: 4.64 [4.11–5.25] Childhood: 1.41 [0.97–2.04] Mortality Risk due to suicide: 8.63 [6.27–11.88] Mortality Risk due to unintentional injury: 3.94 [2.49–6.25]
Chen et al. (2019) Taiwanese nationwide cohort study	275 980 ADHD individuals and 1 931 860 without ADHD	ADHD (relative to controls) All-cause mortality: HR [95% CI] (p) 1.42 (1.31–1.54) (<0.001) Suicide: 3.19 [2.56–3.97] (<0.001) Unintentional injury: 1.21 [1.03–1.41] (<0.01) Homicide: 2.04 [1.13–3.70] (0.007) Natural causes: 1.30 (1.17–1.45) (0.001)

CD, conduct disorder; CI, confidence interval; HR, hazard ratio; MRR, mortality rate ratio; ODD, oppositional defiant disorder; SUD, substance use disorder.

Further reading

Boland, B., DiSalvo, M., Fried, R. et al. (2020). A literature review and meta-analysis on the effects of ADHD medications on functional outcomes. *Journal of Psychiatric Research* 123: 21–30.

Chang, Z., Lichtenstein, P., D'Onofrio, B.M. et al. (2014). Serious transport accidents in adults with attention-deficit/hyperactivity disorder and the effect of medication. *JAMA Psychiatry* V71 (3): 319–325.

Chen, V.C., Chan, H.L., Wu, S.I. et al. (2019). Attention-deficit/hyperactivity disorder and mortality risk in Taiwan. *JAMA Network Open* 2 (8): e198714. https://doi.org/10.1001/jamanetworkopen.2019.8714.

Dalsgaard, S., Østergaard, S.D., Leckman, J.F. et al. (2015). Mortality in children, adolescents, and adults with attention deficit hyperactivity disorder: a nationwide cohort study. *Lancet* 385: 2190–2196.

Faraone, S.V., Banaschewski, T., Coghill, D. et al. (2021). The World Federation of ADHD international consensus statement: 208 evidence based conclusions about the disorder. *Neuroscience and Biobehavioural Reviews* 128: 789–818.

HMICFRS (2021). Neurodiversity in the criminal justice system: a review of evidence. http://justiceinspectorates.gov.uk/hmicfrs/publications/neurodiversity-in-the-criminal-justice-system

Schiavone, N., Virta, M., Leppämäki, S. et al. (2022). Mortality in individuals with childhood ADHD or subthreshold symptoms – a prospective perinatal risk cohort study over 40 years. *BMC Psychiatry* 22: 325.

Shaw, M., Hodgkins, P., Caci, H. et al. (2012). A systematic review and analysis of long-term outcomes in attention deficit hyperactivity disorder: effects of treatment and non-treatment. *BMC Medicine* 10: 99. https://doi.org/10.1186/1741-7015-10-99.

Sun, S., Kuja-Halkola, R., Faraone, S.V. et al. (2019). Association of psychiatric comorbidity with the risk of premature death among children and adults with attention deficit/hyperactivity disorder. *JAMA Psychiatry* 76 (11): 1141–1149. https://doi.org/10.1001/jamapsychiatry.2019.1944.

Takeda UK (2022). ADHD in the Criminal Justice System: a case for change. https://www.adhdfoundation.org.uk/wp-content/uploads/2022/06/Takeda_ADHD-in-the-CJS-Roundtable-Report_Final.pdf

Young, S. (2018). Identification and treatment of offenders with attention-deficit/hyperactivity disorder in the prison population: a practical approach based upon expert consensus. *BMC Psychiatry* 18: 281. https://doi.org/10.1186/s12888-018-1858-9.

CHAPTER 6

An Introduction to Autism

Munib Haroon

OVERVIEW

- Autism is a relatively common neurodevelopmental condition with a prevalence of over 2% in many populations.
- It is a type of neurodivergency with a strong genetic basis, but with a clear contribution from environmental factors.
- Autism is clinically defined by the presence of social communication and social interaction deficits and restricted, repetitive patterns of behaviour, interests or activities, which can vary in presentation.
- Grunya Efimovna Sukhareva wrote the first well-described clinical account of patients with recognisable features of autism in 1926.
- As well as genetic risk factors, there are other maternal/paternal and other environmental factors whose presence can increase the chances of a child being autistic.

Autism (formally autism spectrum disorder) is a relatively common neurodevelopmental condition. It is a type of neurodivergency with a strong genetic basis, but with a clear contribution from environmental factors. How these two factors interact, leading to changes in the developing brain, and how this results in changes in outlook, behaviours and interactions are the subject of ongoing research.

The clinical definition of autism is based on the presence of deficits in social communication and social interaction and restricted, repetitive patterns of behaviour, interests or activities (Figure 6.1). These deficits can vary greatly in severity and, while they are often noticeable during childhood, they may go undetected until later in life.

The neurodiversity movement has had a large impact on the terms of discourse when referring to autism, and for many people use of the term 'autism' is preferred to the terms '… disorder' or '… condition'. In scientific literature, pluralised terminology (e.g. 'disorders') is also often used to highlight the heterogeneous nature of the condition.

The term 'autism' is therefore used preferentially over 'autism spectrum disorder(s)' and 'autism spectrum condition', except on a few occasions in this and the preceding chapters on this topic – for example when referring specifically to guidance/classification schemes. However, for diagnostic purposes, in a clinical setting, it may be preferable to use conventional terminology in a consistent way to avoid confusion.

By definition, autism exists as a spectrum, with what is almost certainly a polygenic pattern of inheritance. As such, the features probably 'blur' into the general population, thus explaining the pattern where many people, for whom a diagnosis would be inappropriate/unnecessary, can still have a few traits of the condition. Despite this, the saying 'We're all a little bit autistic' can often be seen by neurodivergent people as trivialising the issues they can face.

History

The term 'autism' is derived from the Greek word *autos*, meaning 'self', and was first used in 1910 by Eugen Bleuler (Figure 6.2) in relation to schizophrenia, to describe the withdrawal of schizophrenic patients into their own fantasies. However, the earliest clinically based descriptions of what we would now recognise to be autistic patients were not written for many years after this (although there is considerable interest among researchers in older historical descriptions of individuals who seem to possess autistic traits). The first well-described clinical account was written by Grunya Efimovna Sukhareva (Груня Ефимовна Сухарева) in 1926, although credit for the first detailed descriptions of autism are usually attributed to Leo Kanner in 1943 and then to Hans Asperger in 1944. Opinion is divided over which man 'got there first', and who knew what about the others' work – a controversial area whose detailed description lies outside this book's scope. Asperger's contribution to the field fell into neglect in the years surrounding the Second World War before being rehabilitated in 1981 by Lorna Wing, who coined the eponymous term 'Asperger's syndrome'.

ABC of Neurodevelopmental Disorders, First Edition. Edited by Munib Haroon.
© 2024 John Wiley & Sons Ltd. Published 2024 by John Wiley & Sons Ltd.

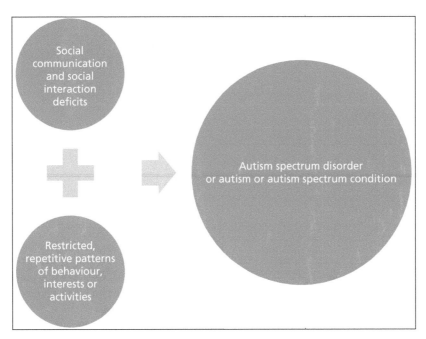

Figure 6.1 Autism is defined by the presence of features in two broad categories.

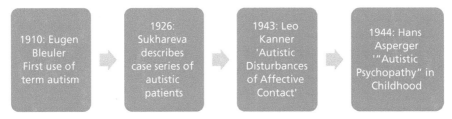

Figure 6.2 A timeline showing some of the early pioneers in autism.

Prevalence

The reported prevalence of autism has increased in recent decades and the previous estimate of a prevalence of around 1% is now felt to be very conservative. In the United States this figure is now 2.3% and in the United Kingdom it has been estimated to be as high as 3% in children and young people.

It is not yet clear how much of this increase could be due to an actual increased incidence, as a large part is likely to be due better public awareness, improved recognition by professionals and a widening of the diagnostic criteria.

Large-scale studies have shown that autism affects two to three times more males than females. This is likely to be due to under-recognition in females, but there may also be a genuine sex difference.

It is likely that autism is under-diagnosed, particularly in adults (especially older ones), and this probably applies even more in females.

Aetiology

Controversy over the aetiology has dogged the condition from early on. It was seen – erroneously – by some as an acquired condition due to parent–child interactions, with 'blame' in some quarters attached to 'refrigerator mums', a theory that was popularised in the 1950s by Bruno Bettelheim. The 1960s saw a shift from 'nurture-based' explanatory models towards 'nature-based' models and towards undertaking research to address the biological basis for the condition. This biological basis remains incompletely understood.

What is clear is that there is a strong genetic basis for autism (along with a clear role for environmental risk factors). It has been known for some time that a sibling of an affected individual is more likely to have autism than a member of the general population (~20% in comparison to 2%). Furthermore, the risk for a monozygotic twin is greater than the risk for a dizygotic twin. More recent research has identified that there are multiple candidate genetic mutations, many of which are uncommon or rare, and their interactions may play a significant role in how the autistic phenotype is expressed. It is likely that the majority of causes are due to the combination of many common 'low-risk' genes (of which there may be thousands), while a minority of cases can occur in the presence a smaller number of 'high-risk' genes.

It is thought that the non-genetic risk factors that have been identified may have an interaction with genetic factors and thus affect how a phenotype is expressed in an individual. Factors that may affect the health and well-being of a mother during pregnancy (gestational diabetes, pre-eclampsia, being overweight) have been identified as contributing to the risk of developing autism, as has the use of sodium valproate in pregnancy and older maternal and paternal ages. Other environmental factors include exposure pre/post-natally to environmental toxins in the forms of air pollutants, heavy metals, herbicides and infections.

Some of the work looking at risk factors has not been without controversy, most notably the well-publicised scare over a study (published in and subsequently retracted by *The Lancet*) that erroneously showed an association between the measles, mumps and rubella (MMR) vaccine and autism, and led to a significant decline in immunisation rates in the United Kingdom in the early twenty-first century. Claims of such an association are refuted by a significant body of research.

Classification

Current classification schemes

Over time, several different classification schemes for autism and related disorders have been proposed, but the two most widely used are from the American Psychiatric Association's *Diagnostic and Statistical Manual of Mental Disorders* (DSM), which is now in its fifth edition (with a text revision in 2022; DSM-5-TR) and the World Health Organization's International Classification of Diseases, which is currently in its eleventh iteration (ICD-11).

DSM-5-TR

Used widely in the United States (but also in Europe, including in the United Kingdom) and updated in 2022, the DSM-5-TR classification uses the overarching term 'autism spectrum disorder' instead of the terminology from the fourth edition of the DSM, 'pervasive developmental disorders'. This single term now replaces the older sub-classifications (e.g. 'autism', 'Asperger's syndrome' 'pervasive developmental disorders not otherwise specified' [PDD-NOS]), with the aim of allowing for more consistent use of terminology by clinicians and researchers, but with the idea that someone previously diagnosed with Asperger's syndrome (a term no longer used in clinical practice in general) would be considered in the newer classification to have an autism spectrum disorder (Figure 6.3). The concept of the clinical heterogeneity seen in autism is represented

not only in the use of the term 'spectrum', but also in specifiers that indicate severity and associated features.

In addition to these changes, the concept of autism as a condition whose core features exist as a 'triad of impairments' (social interaction deficits; social communication deficits; restricted, repetitive patterns of behaviour, interests or activities) has been re-termed a dyad by merging the first two components into social communication and social interaction deficits, because of the recognition that the two components are inextricably interlinked (Figure 6.4).

For those who have social deficits without the restricted, repetitive behavioural elements, a separate criterion for 'social communication disorder' has been developed under which such individuals should be considered, and this may incorporate some of those who would previously have fallen under the PDD-NOS term.

According to the classification a diagnosis is made in the presence of sufficient features affecting the dyad, which cause clinically significant impairments in activities of daily living, whose features have been present since early developmental life (although these may be masked by learned strategies or intellectualisation or may not become apparent until demands exceed native ability) and are not better explained by intellectual disability or global developmental delay. Once a diagnosis is made, DSM allows for a number of modifiers to be made to a standalone diagnosis of autism spectrum disorder. This includes specifying how much support is required, whether there are intellectual and language impairments and stating if there is the presence of other medical, genetic, neurodevelopmental, psychiatric or behavioural conditions or environmental factors (Figure 6.4).

ICD-11

The ICD-11 also uses the term 'autism spectrum disorder'. A diagnosis requires the presence of persistent deficits in social communication and reciprocal social interaction, as well as persistent restricted, repetitive and inflexible patterns of behaviour, interests or activities that are clearly atypical or excessive for the individual's age and sociocultural context. Features should be typically present from early childhood and the diagnosis can be accompanied with relevant specifiers that are designated their own diagnostic codes.

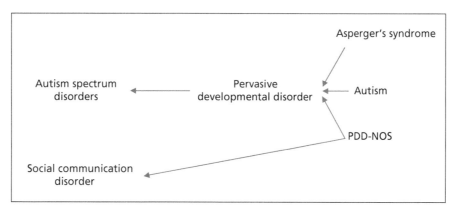

Figure 6.3 In DSM-5-TR the term 'autism spectrum disorder' has replaced 'older' terms such as pervasive developmental disorder and Asperger's syndrome. PDD-NOS, pervasive developmental disorder not otherwise specified.

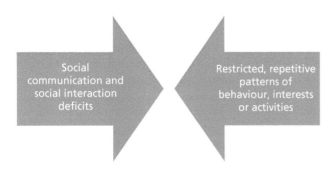

Figure 6.4 The DSM-5-TR classification of autism spectrum disorder is based on the presence of features affecting the 'dyad' since early in development, which are clinically significant and for which there is not a better explanation. The scheme allows for each element of the dyad to be 'graded' for severity and for specifiers to be attached to the diagnosis.

What does a clinician use? DSM or ICD?

For autism spectrum disorders, both the National Institute of Health and Care Excellence (NICE) and the Scottish Intercollegiate Guidelines Network (SIGN) refer clinicians in the United Kingdom to either DSM or ICD. It is important whichever scheme is used that it is the latest version and that it is used in a consistent manner rather than a mix-and-match approach, and in this regard it is important to consider how this is done within a department to enable clear and consistent communication with patients, families and other professionals. The most recent iterations of these schemes are very similar in terms of terminology.

Asperger's syndrome and pathological demand avoidance

Asperger's syndrome, an oft-used and popular term especially among the autistic community, presented a number of difficulties, not least being the inconsistencies in its application and in differentiating what was Asperger's and what was autism. For this reason the term was removed from use, even before the revelations around Hans Asperger's role in the Nazi euthanasia programme.

In recent years there has been considerable interest in the term pathological demand avoidance (PDA) and its use as a separate diagnosis or as a co-diagnosis alongside that of autism. While it is used by some to describe a range of complex behaviours seen in individuals with autism (and possibly without autism), it is not identified in DSM-5-TR or ICD-11 as an independent syndrome.

It is likely that the term fits a constellation of co-occurring features in autistic people where the presentation is also shaped by certain social, familial and mental health factors (such as the presence of coexisting anxiety disorders, ADHD and oppositional defiance disorder).

Autism in culture

There is increasing awareness of autism worldwide, with more representation in popular culture such as novels and movies, and in TV shows such as *The Good Doctor* and *Atypical*. The difficulty with such representations in general includes not only questions around authenticity but the impossibility of showing the breadth of presentation with just one autistic character. There seems to be a particular skewing towards representing neurodivergent characters with savant skills of a level that are uncommonly seen – this has the potential to create misrepresentation. Modern novels portraying autistic or probably autistic characters include *The Curious Incident of the Dog in the Night-Time* and *The Girl with the Dragon Tattoo*. There has also been a lot of interest in past fictional depictions – such as Sherlock Holmes and Phileas Fogg – around the extent to which they may represent autistic characters.

Perhaps more controversially, there has been a lot of interest in historical figures and the possibility that they might have been autistic. While questions about whether Isaac Newton, Paul Dirac and Lewis Carroll were autistic can be fascinating, and may challenge many of the perceptions that people harbour about autism, there are questions about the validity and ethics of making such historical 'diagnoses' in the absence of the living, consenting person they relate to, and with a partial, often biased picture.

Further reading

American Psychiatric Association (2022). *Diagnostic and Statistical Manual of Mental Disorders*, 5e *Text Revision*. Washington, DC: American Psychiatric Association.

Farmelo, G. (2009). *The Strangest Man: The Hidden Life of Paul Dirac, Quantum Genius*. London: Faber and Faber.

Freeman Loftis, S. (2015). *Imagining Autism: Fiction and Stereotypes on the Spectrum*. Bloomington, IN: Indiana University Press.

Haroon, M. (2019). *ABC of Autism*. Oxford: Wiley.

Hirota, T. and King, B.H. (2023). Autism spectrum disorder. A review. *JAMA* 329 (2): 157–168.

Lai, M.C., Lombardo, M.V., and Baron-Cohen, S. (2014). Autism. *Lancet* 383: 896–910.

Manouilenko, I. and Bejerot, S. (2015). Sukhareva – prior to Asperger and Kanner. *Nordic Journal of Psychiatry* 69: 479–482.

Murray, S. (2008). *Representing Autism. Culture, Narrative, Fascination*. Liverpool: Liverpool University Press.

O'Nions, E., Petersen, I., Buckham, J.E.J. et al. (2023). Autism in England: assessing underdiagnosis in population-based cohort study of prospectively collected primary care data. *Lancet Regional Health-Europe* 29: 100626. doi: 10.1016/j.lanepe.2023.100626.

Pugsley, K., Scherer, S.W., Bellgrove, M.A., and Hawi, Z. (2022). Environmental exposures associated with elevated risk for autism spectrum disorder may augment the burden of deleterious de novo mutations among probands. *Molecular Psychiatry* 27: 710–730.

CHAPTER 7

The Presentation, Assessment and Diagnosis of Autism in Children and Young People

Munib Haroon

OVERVIEW

- The features suggestive of autism can usually be recognised from an early age.
- The core features may not be obvious in younger children; sometimes they may only become noticeable in adolescence, or even adulthood – when new stressors come into play or where social demands exceed a person's abilities.
- It is important to interpret possible autistic features in the context of a child's developmental age and ability.
- The presentation in females can be different to that in males and can lead to diagnostic delay.

First concerns

The symptoms, signs and areas of difference and difficulty seen in autism are protean: there is no single feature pathognomonic of the condition.

The core features of autism (see Figure 7.1) relate to the dyad of differences (social communication/social interaction deficits and restricted, repetitive patterns of behaviour, interests and activities), but in addition to these, autistic children may present with many other generalised/non-specific features – especially at a younger age (e.g. speech delay).

Children may also present with features due to comorbid/associated conditions, such as attention deficit hyperactivity disorder (ADHD), anxiety disorders, mood disorders, epilepsy and developmental coordination disorder. When these are present in a child with undiagnosed autism, and when they are marked, they may mask and make it difficult to pick up on the presence of autistic signs.

Normal development

There is a broad range of normality when it comes to the development of speech and social communication and social interaction skills. It is important that clinicians are able to recognise when development is within the normal range and when it is not following the typically seen pattern of development. Development may be delayed – meaning it is following normal pathways but happening later than expected – or it may be disordered. Both delayed and disordered development can occur together. An appreciation of what is normal (and how broad a term it is) only comes through a lot of experience of working with children of different ages and abilities ('typical' time periods for the development of speech, communication and socialisation skills are shown in Table 7.1).

It is also important to think about what we mean by 'normal' and 'abnormal' from a neurodiversity perspective and consider to what extent so many of the variations from the norm that are often seen as 'abnormal' could be better seen as 'differences'.

What is normal for a child at one age can be abnormal at another age. For example, lack of single-word speech in a 2-year-old would be worrying and could indicate that the child needs to be assessed for autism, whereas it would not be similarly concerning in a 9-month-old child. The very young present additional diagnostic challenges for the clinician. For example, those below 2 years may present with non-specific signs rather than features typically associated with autism; as such, it is difficult to be clear what the minimum age is for making a reliable diagnosis.

Because the features change according to age, it is helpful to consider how autistic children may present in different age ranges – for example pre-school children, school-aged children and older adolescents. There is, of course, a lot of overlap between these groups, and the latter will also have features in common with adults (who are considered in Chapter 9).

Male versus female

There can also be differences in presentation between the sexes: females can often have subtler variations in social communication and social interaction and these may not be picked up by others for many years.

It may be that autistic girls intrinsically have fewer differences in these areas to begin with or as they grow up they learn to 'mask' them (some describe autistic girls as being effective 'social mimics' or 'little philosophers'). There can also be qualitative differences in

---

ABC of Neurodevelopmental Disorders, First Edition. Edited by Munib Haroon.
© 2024 John Wiley & Sons Ltd. Published 2024 by John Wiley & Sons Ltd.

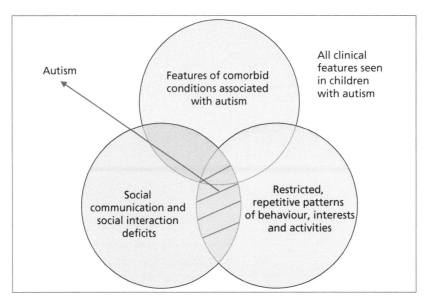

Figure 7.1 There are many clinical features that may be seen in autistic children. The core features of autism relate to those described by the dyad of differences and include social communication and social interaction deficits alongside restricted, repetitive patterns of behaviour, interests and activities. Autistic children will have deficits (or difficulties/differences) in both areas and may also have features associated with other comorbid conditions.

Table 7.1 Speech, communication and socialisation at different ages.

6 months	1 year	18 months	2 years	3 years	4 years
Turns towards familiar voices and listens to voices that are not in view	Responds to own name immediately	Uses 6–20 words and understands many more	Uses 50 or more words Can join 2 words together to form a simple sentence	Modulated speech for loudness and pitch but will still talk to self in monologues	Completely intelligible speech
Looks at and follows parental faces	Babbles with vowels and some consonants Follows the gaze of an adult	Can request using pointing *and* vocalisation and looks to see if an adult has understood	Refers to self by name or 'me' Talks to self in long monologues Repetitive speech	Can reference emotions and show empathy	Understands jokes and has a sense of humour
Recognises facial expressions (e.g. happy)	Plays 'pat-a-cake' and can wave 'bye bye'	Can obey simple instructions – 'hold my hand'	Simple role play Can take turns Plays alongside other children but not with them	Imaginative play including make-believe play with other children Able to share toys	More developed imagination Enjoys dressing up

interests, for example some young autistic girls may be deeply interested in things like animals or dolls – which can easily be passed over as not being relevant to a diagnosis.

Sometimes the person concerned may be aware of these differences as a child, but only begin to place them within a framework of possible neurodiversity when they are an adult and start thinking about the possibility that they may be neurodivergent in some way.

Finally, difference between the sexes in terms of the presentation of comorbid conditions (e.g. ADHD) can compound the difficulty in recognising that a girl or an adult woman needs a referral for further assessment.

Signs of autism in the pre-school child

The features of autism may be noticed from a very young age, although parents are sometimes only able to say in retrospect that

they noticed 'something different' when their child was a baby. And while formal screening for autism in young children is not undertaken in the United Kingdom, it is important that healthcare professionals who work with young children are aware of the signs and features of autism, so that they are able to take appropriate action when they see a child who may require further assessment.

Some of the signs and features associated with autism in the pre-school child are shown in Box 7.1.

Children in whom concerns about autism are raised may show many of these features or only a few, and, as has already been stressed, the signs may not be at all obvious during a short clinical appointment. As such, if there is doubt about what a parent is describing and about the need for further assessment, it will be important to seek further information – for example from the pre-school. This can often be obtained in the form of a report or via the use of an autism-specific screening instrument. Sometimes a longer

Box 7.1 **Signs and symptoms of autism in pre-school children**

- There may be a delay or absence of spoken language. The extent of this can be variable and may become clinically apparent in little time, or may require detailed assessment and exploration to look for alternative causes as well as autism. In older pre-school children, speech patterns that may be normal at an earlier age may persist or stand out, such as repetitive speech or echolalia.
- Children may be reported as not being able to read facial expressions or respond appropriately to them; in a similar vein, they may appear to stare through or past people.
- Eye contact may be unusual: a child may avoid making eye contact or not mesh it in the normal way when using speech, expressions and gestures (e.g. children normally use voice and eye contact to gain a person's attention while they point to an object of interest).
- Aspects of socialisation may differ in a number of ways and encompass variations in showing interest in adults and other children, turn taking, initiating activities such as social play, and sharing toys or other objects of interest and enjoyment. (Girls who are autistic may seem more social than their boy counterparts – at least superficially.)
- Imagination differences may be seen with reduced or absent pretend play.
- Unusual hand/finger or other motor mannerisms such as rocking, spinning or tip-toe walking may be noticeable.
- Changes in routine may lead to children becoming anxious or overly upset – for example, if their route to nursery changes.
- They may have different interests. Young children may not play with toys in the typical way – for example, they may not play imaginatively with action figures, or may only be interested in playing with particular toys (to the point that their play seems to be obsessive), or they may only be interested in parts of toys or other objects, or in lining them up rather than actually playing with them.
- Sensory interests or avoidance of certain sensory stimuli may be particularly noticeable. This can include a dislike of certain sounds (vacuum cleaners, fireworks, children crying) and/or a dislike of tactile (socks, clothes, having hair washed), gustatory and visual stimuli.

period of clinical observation – for example by arranging to see a child for a second time – can also be helpful.

Some of these features may lead to children being described as 'just naughty' by teachers or carers, but while autistic children, like all children, *can* be naughty, it is important not to accept the label of 'naughty' without attempting to scratch beneath the surface. After all, can 'naughtiness' ever really be understood and managed if separated from its underlying cause and explanation?

School-aged children

The features seen in autistic school-aged children can be markedly varied according to their age, their individual personas and the presence of any associated medical conditions. As a child grows, variations noticed during pre-school may persist, become more noticeable or change in character. Sometimes they may become less noticeable over time and may only be prominent during times of stress or transitions (Box 7.2).

Box 7.2 **Signs and symptoms in school-aged children**

- There may be speech abnormalities, which can include ongoing delays in normal development ranging from mild difficulties to a complete absence of speech. Other features of speech often seen include repetitive speech, echolalia; abnormalities of volume, tone, stress or speed; abnormal use of pronouns; or the use of unusual vocabulary including neologisms ('made-up' words) and advanced language. Some children may be reluctant to use speech in a social setting, while others may appear over-garrulous and find it hard to stop talking about certain topics. Speech may appear overly formal and some children are described as 'little professors'.
- Understanding may be different, with some children having a more literal understanding of language and not comprehending sarcasm or metaphors.
- Non-verbal communication, such as the use of eye contact, expression and gesture, may be noticeably different.
- Socialisation differences can include issues with initiating or joining in with others at play or doing other activities. Children may have issues with obeying commonly understood social norms (such as invading the personal space of others, or not tolerating the invasion of their own personal space, or difficulty with being quiet in a library). They may become overwhelmed in groups and display qualitative variations in how they relate to peers or adults – this may include an aversion to such persons or being noticeably over-friendly. Girls may have a subtler presentation and by now have learned to mask some of their difficulties.
- Routines can be important in this age group, as with younger children, although some may hide issues better than others with increasing maturity. Some children's difficulties in managing changes to their routine may not be noticed at home or at school if both environments are themselves rigidly organised and predictable, and it is only when an unexpected change happens (a new supply teacher) or during times of transition (going abroad on holiday, changing school) that the issue is unmasked.
- They may have variations in interests. As with younger children, an autistic child may have normal interests which are abnormally intense (collecting Star Wars figures but *only* Star Wars figures and talking about nothing but); or have somewhat unusual interests for a child of that age (an 8-year-old who is interested in the *Titanic* and knows where it was made, when it sank – down to the precise time – and how many passengers survived), or their interests may be deep but fragmented (they know 'all about' Second World War tanks but not when the war started or why or which countries were involved). In girls a very deep or seemingly 'obsessive' interest in things like animals/pets can easily be missed and passed over as 'something all girls are interested in', but it is the degree of interest that should be picked up on as being unusual.
- Sensory interests can be of a similar nature to those of younger children.

Older adolescents

There is a large amount of overlap between the autistic features described for younger children and those that may occur in adolescent children (Box 7.3). In addition, many adolescents, especially older ones, will have features similar to those seen in adults. As such it is helpful to refer to the information on school-aged children and adults.

Adolescence is marked by hormonal changes and increasing complexity in academic work, social demands – including personal relationships – as well as the pressure of exams, and then, later on, by leaving school and the family home; there are aspects like starting college, university or work. These stressors, which can occur together, can be effective in unmasking what have hitherto been background and unnoticed autistic features, and in triggering associated conditions like anxiety and mood disorders.

History

A detailed history that captures all the relevant information requires an appropriate setting, the right family members/carers to be present, knowing what questions to ask and an appropriate time. It is not something that can be rushed without sacrificing important considerations, and information that is not obtained at the first appointment may have to be sought at a later date; this may lead to delay or additional and unnecessary consultations with the family. Important areas of enquiry are shown in Box 7.4.

The aim of the history (in the context of an autism assessment) is to help determine whether the referred child is autistic or whether there are alternative explanations for their presentation, and also to enquire about possible comorbidities/associated conditions.

An autism-specific tool that relates to the ICD or DSM classifications can be used to supplement a medical history.

Such tools include ADI-R (Autism Diagnostic Interview–Revised), 3Di (Developmental, Dimensional and Diagnostic Interview) and DISCO (Diagnostic Interview for Social and Communication Disorders). All such tools require training and can take a significant amount of time to administer. In children, ADI-R has been shown to be reliable in aiding diagnosis, while data on 3Di suggests that it is comparable in performance to ADI-R.

Examination

The examination is a vital adjunct to the history and requires experience of examining children at different ages and at different stages of development. Autistic children or those with developmental or behavioural difficulties can present with certain challenges (such as severe anxiety leading to non-engagement) and these need to be anticipated and planned for. What cannot be done at the first visit may have to be rearranged for another date, but often a clear and calm explanation in pleasant surroundings with support from a parent/carer who has brought along the child's favourite book or toy and the support of a play therapist can work wonders. It is also important to develop the art of examining a child at a distance – by observing them and seeing how they interact with the environment and their carers.

The purpose of the examination is to tease out autistic features through observation and interaction with the child, and to help think about differential diagnoses/comorbid conditions. It is also an opportunity to examine the child holistically and think about their general health such as growth and nutrition – which may be affected irrespective of a diagnosis of autism. Some areas to think about when examining a child are shown in Box 7.5.

Autism-specific diagnostic instruments can be used to supplement a clinical examination. These include ADOS-2 (Autism Diagnostic Observation Schedule), which provides a reliable and validated way to assess a child and can be completed in approximately an hour. Autism-specific tools such as ADOS-2 and

---

Box 7.3 **Autism can present differently at different ages**

Isaac is 3.5 years old. From a young age his mum noted that he avoided responding to his name and his speech seemed to be delayed – he said no words until he was 20 months. He is very interested in things that spin, such as the wheels on toy cars, fans and the washing machine. He is very mechanically minded but not does enjoy playing with other children, preferring to sit alongside them and play at building towers.

Sally is 7. She appeared to meet all her childhood milestones and seems to be sociable, but her friendships are transient. She is very rulebound and insists that things are done her way, which sometimes causes issues with other children when they disobey the rules of a game. She tends to have just one friend at a time and gets very upset when they play with someone else. She is very dependent on routine and gets upset when there is a supply teacher or when her best friend is off sick. There seem to be no issues at home, where she prefers to spend the majority of her time playing in her bedroom alone and doing maths problems.

Joshua is 17 and currently studying for his A-levels. He is hoping to study Physics at Trinity College, Cambridge. He has always been a very studious boy who has largely kept himself to himself. He has one or two friends who share his interest in science and science fiction. He used to be described as a bully magnet but after studying karate intensely for four years and getting a black belt (which helped his ADHD and dyspraxia no end), he found that the problems largely went away. For the last few months, with approaching end-of-year exams, he has found himself getting obsessed with things being done exactly to plan and getting upset with peers and family members when they seem to obstruct this from happening. He complains about peers being too loud and has sworn and left the classroom. He has always been a faddy eater, but he is eating less and less and has lost 5 kg. His girlfriend has decided that she wants to go to Edinburgh University and he is finding it hard to communicate his distress and is sleeping very badly. He eventually left her a WhatsApp message whose content has not helped the situation.

Box 7.4 **Important points of enquiry when taking a history about possible autism**

- What is the problem and in which settings does it occur? Is it just at home, at school or in multiple settings?
- How do the difficulties affect the child, family and peers?
- Timing: when did the issues begin, are they getting worse?
- Are there any obvious triggers for the difficulties seen?
- Which of the core features of autism are present: are there social communication and social interaction difficulties and repetitive and restricted patterns of behaviour, interests and activities?
- Are there any other associated features such as problems with sleep, seizures, feeding problems, hearing problems, self-injurious behaviours or bowel/bladder problems?
- Are there any features that may suggest comorbid conditions associated with autism, such as ADHD, developmental coordination disorder, depressive disorders, anxiety disorders, obsessive compulsive disorder, tics or Tourette's syndrome.
- The past medical history should include the antenatal history and enquiries should cover the use of maternal alcohol, medication and substance use, as well as asking about the perinatal, birth and neonatal period. Other past medical history should be inquired about – including behavioural and emotional and mental health problems.
- As well as seeking information about any family history of autism, hearing/speech abnormalities or other developmental conditions, it is important to ask about any psychiatric history in the family, such as mood and anxiety disorders, psychosis, obsessive compulsive disorder, bipolar and personality disorders.
- A detailed developmental history asking about delay or regression should be obtained. This can be done using formal developmental tool kits or more informally.
- The social/family history should include asking about the child's education and finding out how they are managing at school, whether they have a learning disability, what supportive structures are employed and whether they have an Education, Health and Care plan. Any current or past involvement with social services (e.g. looked-after status/safeguarding involvement) and the reasons for this are also important to ascertain. Finally, it is important to be clear on the family set-up and what changes have occurred to it in the child's lifetime and why, as well as asking about changes in housing and family employment.

Box 7.5 **Factors to think about when examining a child**

It may not be possible to examine everything at one sitting, and it may not be possible for one professional to assess all of these areas in detail, so where there is suspicion or concern about alternative diagnoses a referral to a relevant service may be required.
- General assessment including growth and nutrition parameters.
- Developmental assessment.
- Assessment for the presence of autistic signs and traits.
- Assessment for the presence of comorbid conditions and other differentials.
- Skin stigmata for neurofibromatosis or tuberous sclerosis using a Wood's light.
- Signs of injury, for example self-harm or maltreatment.
- Congenital anomalies and dysmorphic features including micro/macrocephaly.
- The presence of abnormal neurology, including subtle features and 'soft signs'.

ADI-R should be seen as supplements rather than standalone diagnostic instruments for an autism assessment.

Further adjuncts, which can help to build up a full picture of a child's strengths and difficulties and add context, and which can supplement the assessment, include obtaining information from the school/nursery and other family members and carrying out an observation in a school or home setting. Use of autism-specific tools (e.g. GARS-3, Gilliam Autism Rating Scale) to gather this information can be useful.

Comprehensive assessments of speech/language, communication and assessment of intellectual, neuropsychological and adaptive functioning can also be helpful.

Differential diagnosis and comorbid conditions

A full assessment should allow consideration of whether a child is autistic based on the current ICD/DSM classification schemes (or an alternative diagnosis). Other conditions that might need to be considered as alternative explanations are shown in Box 7.6. In addition, all of these differentials can occur *alongside* a diagnosis of autism along with functional problems involving feeding, sleeping, continence, constipation and visual/hearing difficulties.

Biomedical tests

In general, medical investigations should not be routinely carried out but should be considered on an individual basis, taking into account the presence of dysmorphology, neurocutaneous lesions, congenital abnormalities, intellectual disability and the likelihood of epilepsy. Resource constraints are also an important factor. As well as more traditional investigations such as a comparative genomic hybridisation (CGH) test and Fragile X testing (where felt necessary), whole-genome sequence analysis may need to be considered depending on the clinical presentation.

Other investigations should be carried out for reasons other than to diagnose autism – such as an electroencephalogram (EEG) to confirm a clinical diagnosis of epilepsy or audiology assessments to exclude a hearing impairment.

Box 7.6 **Important differential diagnoses when assessing a child for possible autism**

Neurodevelopmental, mental health or behavioural disorders
- Speech and language delay or disorder
- Intellectual disability
- Global developmental delay
- Traumatic brain injury
- Developmental coordination disorder
- Attention deficit hyperactivity disorder
- Conduct disorder
- Oppositional defiant disorder
- Psychosis
- Depressive disorders
- Anxiety disorders (including selective mutism)
- Attachment disorders
- Obsessive compulsive disorder

Conditions associated with regression
- Rett syndrome
- Epileptic encephalopathy

Other conditions
- Hearing impairment
- Severe visual impairment
- Maltreatment
- Genetic/chromosomal/mitochondrial/disorders, e.g. Fragile X, Williams syndrome, Prader-Willi

Diagnosis

A diagnosis of autism is made, or ruled out, after looking at all of the information gathered and is made in relation to the ICD or DSM classification schemes.

In a child with a sufficient number of chronic features involving the dyad of differences, which are present in more than one setting and are causing functional or other impairments/issues, and where there is not a better explanation, making a diagnosis after the assessments have been completed can be relatively straightforward.

However, occasionally there may be some diagnostic uncertainty. This may occur particularly in those under 2 years, those with a developmental age of <18 months, in children where there is a lack of information about their development (e.g. looked-after/adopted children), older teenagers, or those with a complex mental health disorder, a sensory disorder, cerebral palsy or other motor disorder. In children where a diagnosis is not appropriate but who nevertheless have related or other issues, referrals to alternative services should be considered. Where a diagnosis is unclear but possible, it may be relevant to consider what additional assessments might help, adopting a 'wait-and-see' approach or whether a referral for a second opinion might be useful.

Irrespective of the decision, the outcome of the assessment should be communicated to the carers and where relevant to the patient in a clear, age-appropriate and sensitive manner. While face-to-face feedback has many benefits, a written report should also be prepared, and this should be shared with the GP and with key professionals following parental consent.

Further reading

Haroon, M. (2019). *ABC of Autism*. Chichester: Wiley.

National Institute for Health and Care Excellence (NICE) (2011). Autism spectrum disorder in under 19s: recognition, referral, and diagnosis. [NICE guideline CG128]. https://www.nice.org.uk/guidance/cg128

Scottish Intercollegiate Guidelines Network (SIGN) (2016). Assessment, diagnosis and interventions for autism spectrum disorders. https://www.sign.ac.uk/our-guidelines/assessment-diagnosis-and-interventions-for-autism-spectrum-disorders

Sharma, A. and Cockerill, H. (2014). *Mary Sheridan's from Birth to Five Years*. Abingdon: Routledge.

UK National Screening Committee (2023). A review of screening for autism spectrum disorders in pre-school children under the age of 5 years. https://view-health-screening-recommendations.service.gov.uk/autism

CHAPTER 8

Interventions for Autistic Children and Young People

Munib Haroon

OVERVIEW

- Pharmacological and non-pharmacological interventions do not 'cure' the core features of autism.
- Interventions for autism should be safe, timely, effective, efficient, equitable and patient-centred (STEEEP).
- Pharmacological interventions should be considered as adjuncts to behaviourally based or non-pharmacological interventions.

Questions about interventions, treatment and cures are common following the diagnosis of autism in a child, young person or adult; while there is no shortage of interventions, none is curative or able to remove the core features of the condition. In addition, many interventions have a limited evidence base for beneficial effect (either because of an absence of evidence or a genuine absence of benefit) and some may even be harmful. Some interventions are based on sound, sensible and practical considerations underpinned by an understanding of the difficulties seen in autism, but they may lack a firm evidence base as to their effectiveness.

Many interventions require the input of parents/carers, except where young people are able to act independently. But in order to do this they may need support or signposting from clinicians (Box 8.1), who must have had the right training and know what local services are available. However, hands may be tied if the availability, organisation and delivery of accessible healthcare by suitably trained professionals (see Box 8.2) is not adequately addressed (see Figure 8.1).

High-quality interventions

The Institute of Medicine in the United States (now the National Academy of Medicine) published a report in 2001 that identified six dimensions relating to quality care: safety, timeliness, effectiveness, efficiency, equitability and patient-centredness (STEEEP) (see Figure 8.2). Interventions for autism, whether they are non-pharmacological or pharmacological, and indeed any aspect of healthcare should aim to reflect these parameters. It is important that interventions for autism are done primarily for the health and

Box 8.1 Accurate information on autism and signposting to services

Parents/carers should have access to information on a number of areas:
- The condition itself
- Strategies
- Opportunities to meet others
- Courses
- Welfare benefits/rights
- Education
- Social support
- Leisure
- Treatment
- Transitions
- Short breaks and respite
- How to access help for the broader family

Box 8.2 Adjustments to healthcare to make healthcare more accessible to autistic children and young people

Adjustments to the social and physical environment where children are seen/cared for and to the processes of care must be considered to make healthcare more accessible. Communication may be helped with visual supports (meaningful words, pictures of symbols) and it may be important to think about adjustments to a child's potential personal space and their sensory sensitivities in the ward, waiting room, clinic or treatment room. This may require thinking about seating and the presence/absence of auditory, visual, olfactory and tactile stimuli.

Appointments for autistic children at the start/end of the day may reduce waiting times and issues to do with space/noise or changes to school routine; this may also help with parking. Such changes may be harder to make when running a specific 'autism clinic' where every patient is autistic – but it is still worth thinking about which specific children/young people may benefit most from a first/last approach.

Most people prefer seeing a familiar and friendly professional, but this can be especially the case for autistic children and their families, who especially value routine. Similarly, in the author's experience, children and carers prefer attending a longer neurodevelopmental clinic where multiple conditions can be assessed as opposed to going to separate ADHD/autism clinics.

ABC of Neurodevelopmental Disorders, First Edition. Edited by Munib Haroon.
© 2024 John Wiley & Sons Ltd. Published 2024 by John Wiley & Sons Ltd.

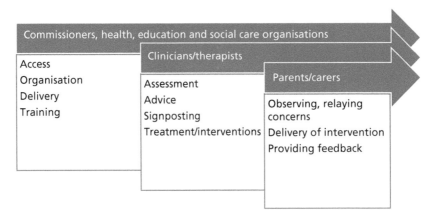

Figure 8.1 Healthcare interventions require the involvement of parents/carers, clinicians and commissioning and related organisations to fulfil a number of roles.

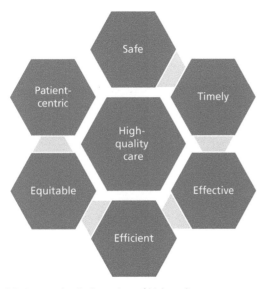

Figure 8.2 STEEEP: the six dimensions of high-quality care.

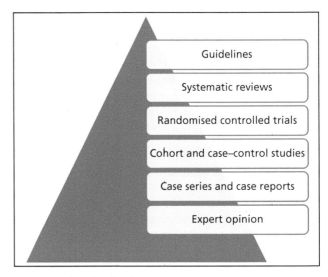

Figure 8.3 Hierarchy of evidence.

well-being and benefit of the autistic person rather than for the sole convenience of those around them.

Evidence-based medicine

Where it exists, evidence about specific interventions for autism and how they address the different dimensions of good-quality care can come from a number of different types of studies or sources (Figure 8.3). Clinical guidelines, such as those issued in the United Kingdom by the National Institute for Health and Care Excellence (NICE) and the Scottish Intercollegiate Guidelines Network (SIGN) that make recommendations on the basis of available evidence, may draw their findings from a hierarchy of clinical studies, although sometimes, where research evidence is not available, recommendations are made on the basis of expert opinion. Expert opinion can either be based on the experience of a Guideline Development Group, using informal consensus processes, or be developed explicitly using formal consensus methodologies such as Delphi panels. Increasingly, guidance and research studies are being designed with the input of autistic people. This involvement should be substantive and not used as a rubber stamp.

Non-pharmacological interventions in children

These range from the simple to the complex; from interventions that can be put in place by parents to those that require ongoing support from professionals. Not every type of intervention will be easily available, because of commissioning arrangements, or worthwhile – when assessed for being of 'high quality'. Occasionally parents will ask whether a particular programme or therapy can be paid for privately. In these circumstances it is important to be realistic and acknowledge the limited evidence for many interventions, so that parents only commit to costly programmes once they are aware of what the potential outcomes may be.

The terms used to describe interventions in the literature can often be broad brush. For example, 'parent-mediated interventions' may be used to describe a variety of programmes with different types of individual interventions administered for differing durations and at various frequencies. In addition, studies may measure different outcomes, or use different tools, on different subsets of autistic children. This clinical and methodological heterogeneity can make it difficult to appraise the literature and come up with generalised recommendations. Where interventions have been shown to lead to improved outcomes, it is then also crucial to ask how long the improvement lasts: an ideal intervention would offer permanent or at least long-lasting benefits.

As a general rule, it is important to consider behavioural interventions before pharmacological ones and to view pharmacological therapies not in isolation but as part of a package of care. As with pharmacological therapy, complex behavioural interventions should be administered by, or led by, people with the necessary experience. The evidence base for such interventions is rapidly evolving and may lead to the modifications of current recommendations made by national bodies like NICE and SIGN.

Interventions can grouped into those that address the core features of autism, interventions for behaviours that challenge, interventions for life skills and interventions for coexisting problems.

Interventions for the core features of autism

In terms of psychosocial interventions, NICE recommends development age-appropriate, play-based strategies with parents, carers, teachers or peers to improve joint attention, engagement and reciprocal communication.

Current evidence shows benefits with models that use behavioural approaches (e.g. early intensive behavioural intervention), developmental approaches (e.g. developmental individual differences) and naturalistic developmental behavioural interventions as well as group social skills interventions. It is important to grasp the idea that trying to change some features may be unhelpful or unpleasant for an autistic person and serve no purpose except to be convenient for those around them. It is important to ask who this helps and why.

Interventions for behaviour that challenges

Parents frequently seek advice about behaviours that they find challenging or behaviours that suggest that a child is experiencing distress. The underlying cause for these should be assessed in a systematic manner considering the causes in Box 8.3. This may require further evaluation in a multidisciplinary setting or liaison with other professionals/senior advice.

In the absence of identifiable medical/mental health or environmental issues, a functional assessment should be done to look for factors that trigger the behaviour, any patterns, what needs

---

Box 8.3 **Possible causes/factors to consider when assessing behaviour that challenges**

- Difficulties with communicating intent to others
- Coexisting physical disorders (e.g. earache, toothache, uncontrolled asthma)
- Coexisting mental health disorders (e.g. anxiety)
- Coexisting neurodevelopmental conditions (e.g. ADHD)
- Physical/social environmental issues
- Changes to routine/circumstances/lack of predictability (new school/teacher)
- Developmental/pubertal change
- Exploitation/abuse/bullying
- Inadvertent reinforcement of behaviours that challenge

---

the child may be trying to meet and the consequences of the behaviour. This will inform any psychosocial intervention.

Psychosocial Interventions should be done systematically, with care taken to address behaviour before and after the intervention, along with the use of clear timescales, agreed and consistently applied strategies, and appropriate outcomes that address quality of life. A very simple example of how a basic intervention could be mapped out is shown in Figure 8.4.

Interventions for life skills

It is important that autistic children and young people have support to enable them to develop practical coping strategies to help them access services that are important for daily living, such as public transport, employment and leisure facilities. It is easy for neurotypical people to take some of these skills for granted. For example, it is easy to assume that an autistic child will grasp the concept of money and time just because they have a very good facility with numbers, but this may not be the case.

Interventions for coexisting problems

Interventions may be required for specific mental health and physical conditions, including neurodevelopmental conditions (see the relevant chapters for details on mental health and other relevant neurodevelopmental conditions). Common conditions encountered in autism include difficulties with sleep (see Box 8.4) and reduced food intake.

Rigidity around foods is very common in children, not just among those on the autism spectrum. In general there is no need to be too concerned if a child is eating foods from each of the main food groups and is growing well. However, advice should be sought if this is not happening; or in the presence of other concerning features such as avoiding food groups; or if a child is presenting with constipation, excessive weight loss/gain, tooth decay, behaviour/clinical features suggesting a nutritional deficiency, signs of aspiration, or they are missing school/social opportunities due to eating problems. There are a number of helpful strategies that can be employed on a proactive basis to help problematic behaviour around food from becoming ingrained or to help with alleviation, especially before it becomes severe and professional input is required (Box 8.5).

Pharmacological interventions in children

As already stated, medication is not curative and has not been shown to improve the core features of autism on the basis of long-term trials. As such, it should be used for managing associated psychiatric and neurodevelopmental comorbidities or for addressing specific and severe behaviours on a short-to medium-term basis (or for treating coexisting medical conditions such as epilepsy). Medication should not be used in isolation, but instead, when required, should form part of a wider package of care.

It should be the *right* medication, at the *right* time, for the *right* child, from the *right* person.

Before commencing medication, it is important to assess what condition or symptoms are being targeted and thus choose an

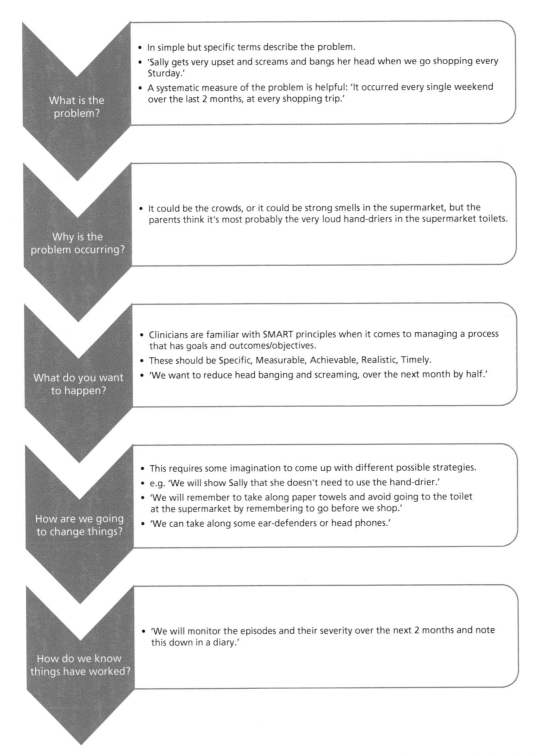

- In simple but specific terms describe the problem.
- 'Sally gets very upset and screams and bangs her head when we go shopping every Sturday.'
- A systematic measure of the problem is helpful: 'It occurred every single weekend over the last 2 months, at every shopping trip.'

What is the problem?

- It could be the crowds, or it could be strong smells in the supermarket, but the parents think it's most probably the very loud hand-driers in the supermarket toilets.

Why is the problem occurring?

- Clinicians are familiar with SMART principles when it comes to managing a process that has goals and outcomes/objectives.
- These should be Specific, Measurable, Achievable, Realistic, Timely.
- 'We want to reduce head banging and screaming, over the next month by half.'

What do you want to happen?

- This requires some imagination to come up with different possible strategies.
- e.g. 'We will show Sally that she doesn't need to use the hand-drier.'
- 'We will remember to take along paper towels and avoid going to the toilet at the supermarket by remembering to go before we shop.'
- 'We can take along some ear-defenders or head phones.'

How are we going to change things?

- 'We will monitor the episodes and their severity over the next 2 months and note this down in a diary.'

How do we know things have worked?

Figure 8.4 Psychosocial interventions should be underpinned by a systematic process to increase the chances of success and so that the effectiveness of the intervention can be determined.

appropriate drug (the right *medication*). The child should be assessed not only in terms of their clinical presentation, but also with respect to their wider circumstances – including those at school and at home – with the aim of seeing if modifications can be made to these areas first (the right *time*). It is important to balance the risks with the benefits of medication, taking into account the child's pre-existing medical history (the right *child*) and to have ensured

that these issues are discussed and understood by the child/patient and carers. It is important to define, as a baseline, which target features the treatment is supposed to address. There should then be a plan for how a child or young person will be monitored and how medication will be managed. Medication should be prescribed by those competent to do so (the right *person*) and with reference to appropriate guidance such as the British National Formulary (BNF).

Box 8.4 **Assessment and management of sleep difficulties in autistic children**

Assessment should address issues such as:
- What is the exact issue: Delay? Early wakening? Night-time behaviours? Day-time sleepiness?
- What is the sleep pattern on a day-to-day basis and during the weekend and holidays? (A sleep diary kept for two weeks will help with this.)
- Sleep environment: is the room shared? Is there any background noise? Are electronic devices used close to bedtime? Are blackout blinds used?
- How much physical activity and exercise is there during the day?
- How is their physical and mental health (e.g. pain, worries, stress, anxiety, bullying)?
- Do they use medication (such as stimulants) and/or caffeine?

Interventions:
- Start by addressing modifying factors seen in the assessment as part of a sleep plan.
- Medication should be used where a sleep plan is not working or where the sleep issues are having a detrimental effect on the child/family (see Table 8.1).
- Referral to a sleep specialist or short breaks/respite care may be required on a case-by-case basis.

Box 8.5 **Helpful mealtime strategies for autistic children**

- Have a regular pattern/time for meals in a regular location.
- Establish a calm and comfortable environment with appropriate table/seating.
- Reduce unnecessary sensory distractions. Music and TV can help but also hinder.
- Sitting with others who are eating helps some children, while others concentrate best when they are not being watched.
- Work to broaden the variety of the diet by initially expanding on already accepted food groups, e.g. different types of breads.
- Try to apply general strategies, e.g. visual supports and positive reinforcement.
- Do not be seen/heard/felt to be stressed as a parent/carer.
- Aim for incremental change. A small bite of something new is a positive step.

Some medications that can be useful and have been shown to be effective for conditions/problems specifically in autistic children are described in Table 8.1.

Table 8.1 Medications with known efficacy in autistic children and young people who have additional healthcare needs.

Second-generation antipsychotics e.g. aripiprizole, risperidone	Can help to reduce irritability and emotional dysregulation Associated with significant side effects that prescribers should be aware of and communicate to carers/patients Effectiveness should be reviewed after 3–4 weeks and medication stopped at 6 weeks if not effective Regular review and a plan for monitoring and shared care are essential Should not be used to manage the core features of autism
Medication for ADHD – methylphenidate, atomoxetine	Medication for ADHD can be very effective and there is evidence from meta-analysis to support the use of methylphenidate and atomoxetine in children with ADHD-type symptoms and autism The evidence for treating children and young persons with other drugs used to treat ADHD is less well founded and should be considered with reference to national guidance, and the BNF, by those experienced in their use
Melatonin	To help with sleep alongside a consistent bedtime routine and sleep hygiene This can be considered in children and young people where there has been an insufficient improvement after behavioural interventions or if necessitated by other clinical factors Medication should be commenced in consultation with a paediatrician or psychiatrist with the relevant expertise, and its use should be appropriately monitored Prescribers/carers/users should be aware of the degree to which melatonin will/will not work

Further reading

Haroon, M. (2019). *ABC of Autism*. Chichester: Wiley.

Hirota, T. and King, B.H. (2023). Autism spectrum disorder. A review. *JAMA* 329 (2): 157–168.

National Institute for Health and Care Excellence (2011). Autism spectrum disorder in under 19s: recognition, referral, and diagnosis. NICE Guideline [CG128]. https://www.nice.org.uk/guidance/cg128

CHAPTER 9

Autism: Adult Considerations

Munib Haroon

OVERVIEW

- The overwhelming majority of autistic people diagnosed in childhood continue to meet the diagnostic criteria as adults.

- Underdiagnosis of autism in adults prevents access to services that could improve quality of life and overall health and well-being.

- Diagnosis of autism is made following a clinical assessment by a qualified professional. There is no role for routine biomedical investigations.

- There are a number of psychosocial and medical interventions available, although it is important to be clear that medication does not reduce autistic traits.

- Autistic adults are less likely to have a full-time job, drive or live independently. Autism is associated with excess mortality due to natural and unnatural causes.

The overwhelming majority of autistic people diagnosed in childhood/adolescence continue to meet the diagnostic criteria in adulthood, although there is evidence that with time a small minority of people no longer meet the diagnosis. The reasons for this observation are not entirely clear and are likely to be complicated. They could include questions over the validity of the original or subsequent diagnosis, a genuine change towards neurotypicality over time, or because the individual learns to mask/camouflage the symptoms with age and experience (Box 9.1). For the majority, however, the core traits of autism (differences in social communication and social interaction alongside restricted, repetitive patterns of activities, behaviours and interests) remain; which makes sense, given the genetic and brain-based features of the condition.

Autism is by definition a condition whose features have been present from childhood; however, a number of people only seek a diagnosis as an adult. There may be a number of reasons for this diagnosis not being made earlier in life (Box 9.2). When adults wonder if their neurodivergent traits may be explained by them being autistic and look back to their childhood, they may identify a number of autistic traits like those described in earlier chapters

(Box 9.3). Some may have always suspected that they might have been autistic. For others, increased awareness following research or exposure to the current cultural milieu, in which autism is a more prominent feature, may have factored in their thinking. Regardless, the subsequent decision on whether to seek a diagnosis will be influenced by the availability of a diagnostic service (or its cost), their concerns around how a diagnosis will be perceived by other people and uncertainty over what benefits a diagnosis will bring. To be or not to be diagnosed is not a simple decision.

However, not getting a diagnosis of autism (which is felt to be underdiagnosed in adults) can prevent access to a diverse range of support, which may affect quality of life and health/well-being–related outcomes. A formal diagnosis can also bring clarity and certainty by way of an explanation for why things have always been the way they have. Nevertheless, some people who see themselves as being neurodivergent or autistic will argue that it does not and should not require seeking a medical diagnosis (through a long, convoluted process) to be able to achieve self-understanding and clarity.

Features of autism in adults

In terms of presentation, autistic adults can share many of the features seen in adolescents, although they may be subtler or less noticeable depending on the autistic traits themselves or because of factors like intelligence, speech ability, or the presence/absence of a syndrome or other comorbidities. They may also be influenced by the environments the adult lives and works in.

Social communication and social interaction difficulties

The range of possible features is broad and the absence of particular traits does not rule out a diagnosis. Similarly, the presence of a few traits does not mean that a person is autistic either – the diagnosis is based on a clinical assessment to determine the presence of sufficient features on both areas of the 'dyad'. These should have been present in some form since childhood and be causing significant issues in areas of life or activities of daily living.

ABC of Neurodevelopmental Disorders, First Edition. Edited by Munib Haroon.
© 2024 John Wiley & Sons Ltd. Published 2024 by John Wiley & Sons Ltd.

Box 9.1 **M on autism, eye contact and masking**

'I still remember when I was a teenager and a classmate very pointedly asked me "why don't you look at me when you're talking to me?" I was quite flustered – I knew I avoided this in general, but I'd never been caught out before. I jokingly said something about how the surroundings were far more visually appealing today, but the truth was that I found making sustained eye contact just "not quite right". As an adult I still don't. It does cause occasional difficulty. But over time I have programmed my mind to remind me to make eye contact with people I'm talking to, even if for a few seconds. I think it works – that, or maybe I've not met anyone else quite like *that* classmate. What you might find to be the strangest thing, however – but maybe it's not at all that strange, actually – is that I am very adept on picking up on very small changes. New earrings, new haircut, a slightly lighter shade of hair – I'll probably notice it. If you're autistic and reading this, I'm not saying that you need to change your behaviours because it may suit other people – sometimes this may be impractical or unpleasant, and you should be accepted for who you are, but it's what I've done for this issue. I suppose that many autistic people do the same, and the point I want to make is how this relates to diagnosis: it makes it a challenge because over time these masking manoeuvres skilfully conceal the traits beneath the surface.'

Box 9.2 **Possible reasons for failure to diagnose autism in childhood**

- Inadequate resources, e.g. paediatric/Child and Adolescent Mental Health Services (CAMHS).
- Other difficulties within the family/child that override concerns about autism, e.g. extremely difficult behaviour or childhood abuse.
- Comorbidities, e.g. learning disabilities, anxiety, obsessive compulsive disorder, genetic conditions.
- Symptoms do not cause a problem in childhood, e.g. 'easy baby'; impeccably behaved, high-achieving student.
- Child shares similar characteristics with their family.
- Child develops coping strategies/masking that hide their social differences.
- Lack of knowledge about autism in the past.

Some women may be especially adept at camouflaging/masking their features or mimicking accepted social norms. They may also be more likely to internalise the processes by which they respond to their perception of being different or of the world around them.

Some of the possible social communication and social interaction features seen in autistic adults are described in Boxes 9.4–9.6.

It is important to stress (if it is not obvious) that while these differences can increase the propensity for two-way miscommunication, there is nothing intrinsically wrong with not making eye contact, nor having a flattened tone, nor being relatively blunt when speaking. A lot of the difficulties encountered by autistic people are problems of perception – how neurotypical people perceive them.

Box 9.3 **Lisa: identifying traits in retrospect**

'As an elementary school student, I rarely approached other children. My main way of play was recreating certain scenes from my favourite cartoons, and I was very particular about following the story exactly as it was in the original. When other children approached me to take part, I generally never refused but would eventually get upset by either them trying to change the story or adding in other characters, which resulted in me choosing to play alone most of the time.

In middle school, I found communication with girls quite difficult. It seemed like there were some kinds of unspoken rules I never came to understand. Girls were generally nice but you had to intuitively understand what they thought about you, if someone didn't like you, why, and what you were supposed to do about it. There was a lot of guessing whether it was alright to approach someone or not when it came to seeking cooperation.

On the other hand, communication and cooperation with boys was a lot easier to achieve. Boys seemed to be less nice towards me, but if someone didn't like you or if you did something wrong, they'd let you know, which made it easier to understand who you could approach when you needed to and how to behave appropriately'.

Often the problem that brings adults (and young people) to clinic is not the actual differences, but the long-term effects of not been accepted for who they and the results of stigma, stereotyping, discrimination and marginalisation.

It can be helpful to adopt the neurodiverse viewpoint of seeing difficulties in social communication/interaction between neurotypical and neurodivergent people as arising because of a two-way difference: like a Spanish speaker and an Urdu speaker trying to strike up a conversation on meeting in a third country (where neither can insist on their way being the right way to communicate).

Restricted, repetitive patterns of behaviour, interests or activities

Some of the issues seen in early or later childhood may be totally absent by the time a person reaches adulthood (many stereotyped movements are typically features of early childhood, like spinning and flapping). Or if present they may be masked and only displayed in certain environments (when relaxed and at home, for example) or become apparent during times of stress. For instance, they may retreat into the reassurance of an additionally rigid routine in the face of uncertainties or take a even greater interest in what may be otherwise less noticeable preoccupations. Some of the features that may be seen in adults with autism are shown in Box 9.7.

Assessment and diagnosis of autism

Similar principles apply as those for children and young people. A team-based comprehensive assessment (history and observation) should be carried out, drawing on evidence from the person seeking assessment as well as from a family member/carer/partner. Assessment should look for core features of autism but also address

Box 9.4 **Differences in use and understanding of verbal and non-verbal language**

- *Gestures* may seem exaggerated, not in keeping with the content of the conversation or very limited/absent relative to neurotypical norms.
- *Social gaze* is often different. The classic absence of eye contact in childhood is often missing in adulthood – due to the repeated instructions from parents or teachers 'to look at people when talking to them' – but the quality of eye contact may be fleeting or unusually even (due to a lack of social instinct some people time/count how long they hold the gaze and then look away as they cannot work this out naturally).
- *Facial expressions* may be incongruous – smiling/laughing when telling a sad story, a fixed grin or an expression that gives no indication of how they are feeling.
- *Tone of voice* may be flatter than neurotypical norms and described as monotonous, or of unusual pitch (high or low), or the person may speak with an American accent (learned from Disney films) despite living in the United Kingdom.
- *Jokes* may be occasionally tried out in inappropriate settings and there may be difficulty understanding some forms of humour (when non-literal understanding of language seems to be an issue). Sometimes jokes may be misconstrued as racist or sexist etc., but they may also have an excellent sense for slapstick and be adept with puns and wordplay.
- *Sarcasm and irony* can be difficult to understand – and may be taken literally. Literal interpretations can cause other problems – e.g. an employer suggesting sarcastically 'You might as well go home if that's the type of work you're going to do' but not really wanting them to leave.
- *No or fairly limited speech* – some autistic people choose not to communicate using speech or have little usable speech. In these circumstances never underestimate how much they understand. Just because they do not speak does not mean they do not understand exactly what you are saying.

Box 9.5 **Language difficulties that may be seen in an adult with autism**

- *Altered prosody* – i.e. the typical up-and-down intonation that implies meaning can be missing, and the variability of voice may be described by some as computer-like and mechanical. In some cases, language and phrases have been learned from TV and films and therefore the accent may seem incongruent and unexpected given their heritage.
- *Language development* – the history in the medical notes may suggest variant or delayed language, or conversely unimpaired or even advanced language development. In adulthood there can be language problems, but even where language is not delayed the use of speech does not seem normal – e.g. abnormally complex language when the situation does not demand it or making repeated subtle grammatical errors out of keeping with their intellectual ability.
- *Echolalia* – repetition of speech. This may be subtle, with the autistic person merely repeating the last couple of words that have been said, as if in acknowledgement. It may be accompanied by *echopraxia*, where the adult is copying the gestures or actions of the person interacting with them.
- *Pronominal reversal* – autistic adults may have difficulty using pronouns correctly when referring to themselves, e.g. using he or she instead of I.
- *Use of third person* – autistic adults may refer to themselves in the third person, i.e. using their own name when talking about themselves. Some research suggests this may not just be a language issue but could be related to their concept of self.
- *Other language anomalies* – there are many similarities with speech disorder seen in mental health conditions such as schizophrenia, which may cause confusion and incorrect diagnosis. Adults with autism may use their own jargon or idiosyncratic and unusual terms (neologisms). Their speech may be tangential, 'wordy' and they may verbalise every thought in a running commentary.

childhood development, additional behavioural and functional issues and the contexts and environments in which they occur (home, education, work, recreation). Assessment should look for coexisting mental and physical conditions and other neurodevelopmental conditions. The possibility of self-harm or risk to others should also be assessed, as should the presence of challenging behaviour.

Documentary evidence such as school reports can be invaluable, and formal assessment tools such as ADI-R, ADOS-2 or DISCO (among others) can be helpful. (See previous chapters for more information on these tools.)

Biological or genetic testing or neuroimaging is not recommended routinely by the National Institute for Health and Care Excellence (NICE).

Interventions

As with children, having effective commissioning and care arrangements that involve all relevant professional groups is important, as is having appropriately trained professionals who carry out these interventions.

Similarly to autistic children, it is important to think about the environment when working with autistic adults. This includes considering their personal space, the use of visual supports, paying attention to distracting elements in the immediate vicinity such as sound, lighting, the colouring and pattern of walls and carpets and the duration of assessments. Evaluating the effectiveness of many interventions remains difficult as much of the evidence comes from children and young people.

Box 9.6 **Examples of differences in social interaction**

- Difficulty in social relationships. It may have been hard to make friends and keep them. In clinic, ask about friendships at school and college. Have they kept in touch? Do they have friends now who they meet up with (including online friends)? Autistic people may relate much better to other autistic people.
- There often seems to be a history of being bullied at school.
- Difficulty with social cues – there may be a tendency to stand too close, to keep talking when the listener is clearly not interested or trying to leave.
- Difficulty understanding and predicting other people's intentions and behaviour.
- Difficulty imagining situations that are outside their own routine, i.e. differences in social imagination (but equally so, autistic adults may be very creative).
- Difficulty fully recognising and understanding people's feelings and managing their own feelings.
- Can cause offence without intention due to a lack of understanding – e.g. if someone asks their opinion on an outfit they tell the truth. (It is important to note that adults, especially women, with autism may have learned not to give an opinion when asked so as not to make a faux pas.)
- Failure to recognise neurotypical emotional cues – they may not notice when someone is upset and may not provide the required comfort (not due to lack of caring, but out of lack of awareness of what is wanted of them).
- Atypical expression/response – e.g. laughing at sad news.
- Atypical interpretation of a situation.
- Problems with personal organisation and time management, which may also have impacts on social relationships.
- Paucity of conversation, or unusual flow of talking or content, or unconventional back and forth of conversation.

Box 9.7 **Restricted, repetitive patterns of behaviour, interests or activities**

- Stereotyped/restricted motor movements, object use or speech. Some adults stop lining up toys but line up other objects, or may continue to rock their body when they require reassurance. Sometimes they may echo a particular phrase (for example, a word that feels 'nice' or amusing) or use idiosyncratic phrases.
- A need for sameness and routines and ritualised behaviour and language may be prominent. Autistic people may not have the same degree of flexibility and may be 'thrown' by small changes or when their routine cannot be kept. They may like to take the same route to work, park in the same spot, and then greet other people in exactly the same way for no other reason than that they like the routine.
- They may have very restricted or fixed interests that are characterised by a great intensity/focus or their seemingly idiosyncratic nature. This may be an academic interest that becomes part of their job or a side interest/hobby; it may be related to objects (cars) or theories (particle physics). This may lead to great expertise in a field. It may become apparent during social interactions, which can be driven by the person talking at great length about their particular 'pet' topic.
- Sensory hyper/hypo-reactivity. This may be in relation to any of the senses. Some autistic people have altered thresholds for pain, they may be distressed by sounds that others would not notice, they may be particularly affected by certain textures and tastes or visual phenomena (adversely or pleasurably), and this may in turn affect outward manifestations of behaviour and even how they take part in activities of daily living.

Several different interventions are available depending on what issues are being addressed. In the United Kingdom further guidance is available from NICE. These may be to address the core features of autism, challenging behaviour or other associated comorbid conditions: physical, mental or neurodevelopmental. Interventions should be identified on a needs- and ability-based assessment. For example, suitable programmes may vary according to the presence/absence of intellectual disability and the extent to which a person is happy in a group-based environment (Figure 9.1 gives further details). While medication may be used to treat associated medical/psychiatric/neurodevelopmental conditions or challenging behaviours, there is no medication that can reduce the core features of autism.

Living with autism

Language skills and cognitive abilities in childhood seem to be good predictors of independence, and of better outcomes for education and employment, although even with high levels of these abilities, autistic adults may look back at life and report a sense of not having achieved their potential. On average, autistic adults are less likely to have a full-time job, live independently or have a driving licence compared to neurotypical people; while some autistic adults would be entirely content not to work full-time or to drive, these outcomes suggest the presence of a disparity in opportunity and outcome. This may occur due to a combination of biological and societally mediated reasons.

Autism is a neurodevelopmental condition that often co-occurs with other conditions (for instance alongside ADHD and

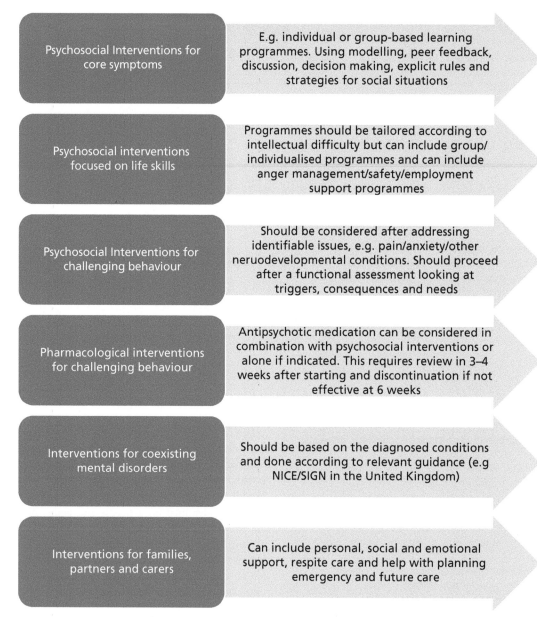

Figure 9.1 There are a number of intervention available for autistic adults. These should be based on the best available evidence. Given the broad spectrum of presentation and the variations in comorbid features, especially intellectually disability and mental health conditions, not every intervention will be required or appropriate for every individual. It is important to note that medications do not help with the core features of autism. NICE, National Institute for Health and Care Excellence; SIGN, Scottish Intercollegiate Guidelines Network.

intellectual disability). In addition, autistic adults may have a range of mental and physical health conditions like epilepsy or anxiety and mood disorders. All of these can pose issues with long-term health outcomes and can impinge on certain aspects of day-to-day life. *Some* autistic adults may come from disadvantaged backgrounds and have experienced adverse life events in childhood, been in a care setting or experienced trauma. Many autistic adults grow up having faced misunderstanding, stigma, discrimination and bullying over many years, in multiple settings, and this overshadows their lives for a long time. It is also possibly a major determinant for whether they will develop mental health difficulties in the first place.

Studies have consistently shown an increased likelihood of early death in autistic people. One study suggested that on average autistic people may die 16 years earlier than the general population and individuals with autism and a learning disability may die on average 30 years earlier. A 2022 meta-analysis of 12 studies found that all-cause mortality in autistic individuals was increased in both sexes with a risk ratio of 2.37 (95 confidence interval [CI] 1.97–2.85). It was noted that in autistic people, deaths from both 'natural' and 'unnatural' causes were increased. The association between autism and unnatural death has also been noted in a number of other studies, which have found increased rates of suicide in autistic people compared to the general population.

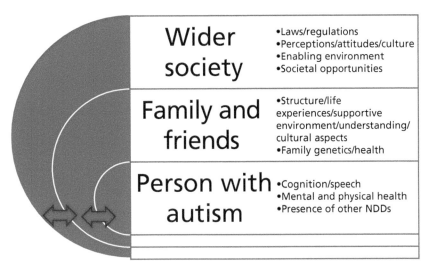

Wider society	•Laws/regulations •Perceptions/attitudes/culture •Enabling environment •Societal opportunities
Family and friends	•Structure/life experiences/supportive environment/understanding/cultural aspects •Family genetics/health
Person with autism	•Cognition/speech •Mental and physical health •Presence of other NDDs

Figure 9.2 While language skills and cognitive abilities are recognised as being good predictors of independence and good educational outcomes and employment, there are likely to be many factors that have a bearing on how well an autistic person can maximise their potential for leading a fulfilling life. This is probably down not just to innate issues like mental and physical health (which themselves may be affected by the presence of wider factors, like quality of care or the effect of bullying), but also to aspects like living in a supported, predictable environment, which may be influenced by the experiences of other family members (which may in turn be influenced by both nature and nurture). It will also be affected by wider aspects of society like laws, attitudes, how supportive environments like school and work are, and by the general opportunities present in a society, which will vary from country to country and be dependent on politics, economics and technology. NDDs, neurodevelopmental disorders.

Conclusion

There is much that needs to be addressed to fully support autistic adults and their families and loved ones to mitigate against the challenges that can occur from societal marginalisation, difficulties in accessing healthcare and the presence of mental and physical health difficulties. Addressing all of these is not down to healthcare alone (Figure 9.2), but earlier diagnosis and treatment of health-related issues and access to appropriate interventions would be welcome, and so would access to reasonable adjustments at school, university, college and work (and being able to tweak things appropriately at home too). Some of this is also about everyone in society having a better understanding and appreciation for autism: what it is and what it is not. It is also about having appropriate support in place, not just from the organisations that matter but from the people who matter as well (Box 9.8).

Box 9.8 On friendship

'I don't want to generalise, but I don't think that what I am going to say is an "n = 1 phenomenon". Autistic people may have experienced difficulties in making friends, especially with neurotypical people, and when they do make friends they may be fewer in number. But quantity ≠ quality, right? That's not to say that friendship doesn't matter to us. It does.

And I have to say that since making friends with another autistic person, I've discovered just *how* important friendship is for me. They're good for my well-being and are a conduit for finding and developing interests and discussing what matters to me (with a likeminded non-judgemental person). Sure, I love my family as much as anyone else, but when you meet someone who has had so many of the same experiences ("What you too?! Why am I not surprised!"), who thinks like you, and makes you realise that you aren't an n = 1 random event in a strange cosmos. . . it. . . just kinda all falls into place.'

Further reading

Catala-Lopez, F., Hutton, B., Page, M.J. et al. (2022). Mortality in persons with autism spectrum disorder or attention-deficit/hyperactivity disorder a systematic review and meta-analysis. *JAMA Pediatrics* 176 (4): e216401. https://doi.org/10.1001/jamapediatrics.2021.6401.

Haroon, M. (2019). *ABC of Autism*. Chichester: Wiley.

Hirota, T. (2023). Autism spectrum disorder. A review. *JAMA* 329 (2): 157–168. https://doi.org/10.1001/jama.2022.23661.

Kölves, K., Fitzgerald, C., Nordentoft, M. et al. (2021). Assessment of suicidal behaviors among individuals with autism spectrum disorder in Denmark. *JAMA Network Open* 4 (1): e2033565. https://doi.org/10.1001/jamanetworkopen.2020.33565.

National Institute for Health and Care Excellence (2011). Autism spectrum disorder in under 19s: recognition, referral, and diagnosis. NICE guideline [CG128]. https://www.nice.org.uk/guidance/cg128

O'Nions, E. (2023). Autism in England: assessing underdiagnosis in a population-based cohort study of prospectively collected primary care data. *Lancet Regional Health – Europe* 29: 100626.

Pickles, P., McCauley, J.B., Pepa, L.A. et al. (2020). The adult outcome of children referred for autism: typology and prediction from childhood. *Journal of Child Psychology and Psychiatry* 61 (7): 760–767. https://doi.org/10.1111/jcpp.13180.

CHAPTER 10

An Introduction to Intellectual Developmental Disorders

Munib Haroon and Keri-Michèle Lodge

OVERVIEW

- Intellectual developmental disorders (IDDs) are conditions that occur when the brain is developing and affect intellectual and adaptive functioning/performance.
- Children may present with global developmental delay alongside or before the IDD is evident.
- IDD may be caused by innate biological/genetic factors or environmental factors or an interaction between them.

The term 'intellectual developmental disorder' (IDD) refers to conditions (see Box 10.1 for an example) whose onset occurs during the developmental period of the brain (which continues for at least two years after birth). They can affect intellectual and adaptive functioning and performance (see Box 10.2).

Children with IDD may present with global developmental delay before it is possible to accurately determine the level of intellectual development and adaptive function (although this is not always the case). The term 'global developmental delay' is used where children under the age of 5 are significantly delayed in two or domains of

---

Box 10.1 A boy with an intellectual developmental disorder

John, 5 years old, has been referred to a paediatric department for further assessment. He has been seeing speech and language therapists who are concerned that his delay is more global than first thought. John has difficulty with expressing speech but also with understanding, dressing and motor movements. His school has arranged for him to be seen by an educational psychologist. John was born prematurely at 36 weeks' gestation; there was concern about sepsis because of a maternal fever and he was treated with intravenous antibiotics, although blood cultures were negative. His father had an Education, Health and Care plan (EHCP) and his paternal uncles both went to special schools.

Box 10.2 Examples of intellectual and adaptive functioning

Intellectual functioning/performance (should be based on clinical assessment but also based on standardised norm-referenced intelligence testing):
- Processing information
- Learning facts
- Learning from experience (applying rules to newer situations)
- Making inferences and deductions
- Abstract learning

Adaptive functioning/performance (looking across different domains such as home, school, work, clubs):
- Self-care skills, such as washing, dressing and eating, telling the time and using money
- Communication (verbal and non-verbal)
- Social engagement, including making and maintaining friendships

---

childhood development, which include gross and fine motor functioning, speech/language and personal/social functioning. Examples of typical attainment are shown in Table 10.1. It is important to note that there can be a wide range of normality. For example, children may not normally take their first steps until 18 months of age and so failing to meet the parameters in Table 10.1 is not a reason for alarm.

As they get older, start school and reach the age at which intellectual functioning can be reliably tested, children with persisting global developmental delay should be diagnosed with IDD (although this may not always happen). When a diagnosis of global developmental delay is changed to a diagnosis of IDD, the child's parents or carers should be kept informed of their child's diagnosis so that they can access appropriate information and support. In general, children with more severe developmental delays in more areas of development are more likely subsequently to be diagnosed with IDD. Developmental delays that are milder and affect fewer areas of development may not be predictive of later IDD.

Table 10.1 Typical developmental parameters for motor, speech/language and personal/social development.

Age	Motor	Speech/language	Personal/social
6 months	Rolls front to back Palmar grasp	Monosyllabic babble	Generally friendly with strangers Can share focus of play with a toy
1 year	First steps Pincer grasp	Understands simple instructions Vocalises a few words	Waves 'bye bye' Drinks from a lidded cup
2 years	Runs Imitates a drawn vertical line	Joins two words together in speech Follows two-step instructions	Plays alongside other children Simple solitary make-believe
3 years	Walks up stairs, one foot per step Copies a drawn circle	Asks 'what', 'where', 'who' type questions Counts to 10	Joins in make-believe with other children
4 years	Hops Copies a cross	Counts to 20 Enjoys simple jokes	Likes dressing-up Shows concern for other children in distress
5 years	Walks along a line Copies a square (copies a triangle at 5.5 years)	Can state name, age, birthday and maybe address Fluent speech Uses abstract terms	Dresses and undresses alone

In some countries, the terms 'IDD' and 'intellectual disability' are used synonymously with 'learning disability'. These terms have superseded the term 'mental retardation', which is now considered derogatory. However, terminology varies between educational and health settings, and there can be confusion between 'learning disability' and 'learning difficulty' (see Box 10.3).

It is estimated that 2.7% of school-aged children and 2.17% of the adult population in England have an IDD, while 1–3% of children 5 years or under have global developmental delay.

The severity of IDD can be classified as mild, moderate, severe and profound (see Table 10.2).

Although this classification system can give a general indication of a person's likely abilities, it should be noted that each individual will have their own unique strengths and needs (Box 10.4). Indeed,

Box 10.3 **Terminology**

Learning disability refers to global impairment of intellectual functioning and adaptive functioning.

Learning difficulty informally refers to a specific difficulty within a particular area of learning, but one in which global intelligence and functioning is not impaired. Formally this is classified as 'specific learning disorder'. Examples include:
- Dyslexia (characterised by specific difficulties with reading and spelling).
- Dyscalculia (characterised by difficulties understanding numbers and calculating).
- Dysgraphia (characterised by difficulties with writing and organising).

Table 10.2 Characteristics associated with different severities of intellectual developmental disorder (IDD).

Severity	Proportion of total IDD population (%)	Approximate intelligence quotient (IQ) range	Approximate adaptive functioning
Mild	85	50–69	Difficulties may be more subtle and diagnosis may be missed in childhood Likely to have difficulties with academic work May be able to maintain some friendships May require only minimal support with daily living skills, such as brushing teeth, washing, dressing In adulthood, may be able to live independently or with minimal support
Moderate	10	35–49	Language and communication skills often adequate to communicate their needs May be able to learn some daily living skills In adulthood, will need varying levels of support
Severe	3–4	20–34	Likely to have significant language delay and difficulties communicating with others Likely to have marked impairment of fine and gross motor skills May be able to complete simple tasks under supervision, but in adulthood likely to need continuous support
Profound	1–2	<20	Severely impaired communication May struggle to communicate their needs Often associated with restricted mobility, incontinence and very limited self-care abilities In adulthood, require continuous care and support Disorder may be associated with hearing and/or visual impairment and epilepsy

Box 10.4 **Clinical tip**

When communicating with a child with possible IDD, do not make assumptions about their level of receptive and expressive communication. They may be able to understand more than they can express. Clinicians should adjust their communication style to ensure that they speak to the child (not just their family/carers) and include them in consultations.

Table 10.3 Categorisation of intellectual developmental disorder according to timing.

	Example
Prenatal	Chromosomal and genetic anomalies: Down's syndrome (Trisomy 21), Fragile X syndrome, copy number variants
	Errors of metabolism/enzyme deficiencies, e.g. phenylketonuria, Lesch–Nyhan syndrome
	Neurocutaneous syndromes: neurofibromatosis, tuberous sclerosis
	Non-genetic congenital malformations: microcephaly, hydrocephalus
	Congenital infections: TORCH infections (toxoplasmosis, rubella, cytomegalovirus, herpes simplex and herpes zoster), Zika virus, syphilis
	Congenital hypothyroidism
	Substance use in pregnancy, e.g. alcohol
	Exposure to teratogens, e.g. prescribed medication such as sodium valproate, lead, radiation
Perinatal	Prematurity, e.g. intraventricular haemorrhage, hyperbilirubinaemia
	Birth trauma, e.g. hypoxic-ischaemic encephalopathy
	Infections
Postnatal	Infections, e.g. meningitis, encephalitis
	Metabolic, e.g. low blood glucose, hyperbilirubinaemia
	Trauma, e.g. accidental or non-accidental head injury
	Exposure to environmental toxins, e.g. lead, mercury
	Hypoxia, e.g. drowning/near drowning
	Severe neglect

it is becoming increasingly common when specifying the severity of IDD to place more emphasis on the level of adaptive functioning rather than the results of intelligence quotient (IQ) tests. This can be helpful, because understanding a person's level of function gives a better idea of what support may be required and what they can do and understand; there is limited professional time to carry out detailed IQ tests; and IQ testing becomes less accurate at the lower end of the IQ range.

Aetiology

The aetiology of IDD is multifactorial, including innate/genetic/medical and environmental causes of disruption to the normal development and functioning of the brain. In a large number of cases, particularly in those with mild IDD, there may not be an identifiable cause. This could occur when an underlying genetic condition has not yet been recognised and described in the literature, or because an environmental insult was transient and thus no longer detectable.

In general, the causes of IDD can be categorised depending on when the causal factor occurred: prenatally, perinatally or postnatally (see Table 10.3).

While alcohol is a well-recognised cause of neurodevelopmental disorder, foetal alcohol spectrum disorder or the DSM-termed 'neurobehavioural disorder associated with prenatal alcohol exposure' has not yet been classified by DSM-5-TR under a particular classificatory heading. Nevertheless, as an increasingly recognised disorder, with neurodevelopmental/behavioural consequences, which could potentially be classed by DSM as an NDD, it will be dealt with in Chapter 24.

Severe neglect resulting in lack of opportunities to learn, such as that experienced by children living in large institutions where they receive little stimulation, is a potentially reversible cause of IDD. Previous studies of children who moved from such institutions to homes where they received adequate care and support showed improvements in IQ up to 20 years later compared to their peers who remained living in the institution.

When a child presents with possible IDD, thorough assessment is needed to identify aetiological factors to enable the child and their family/carers to understand the prognosis, consider genetic testing for other family members and access appropriate support, including peer support. Often aetiological factors coexist, and this is another good reason why children presenting with possible IDD should be assessed carefully.

Further reading

American Psychiatric Association (2022). *Diagnostic and Statistical Manual of Mental Disorders*, 5e. Text Revision. Washington, DC: American Psychiatric Association Pusblishing.

Sharma, A. and Cockerill, H. (2014). *From Birth to Five Years*, 4e. Abingdon: Routledge.

CHAPTER 11

The Assessment and Diagnosis of Intellectual Developmental Disorders in Children and Young People

Munib Haroon and Keri-Michèle Lodge

OVERVIEW

- Children with a suspected intellectual developmental disorder (IDD) may present in a number of different settings, including health and education.
- Determining the presence and potential cause of IDD is vital to ensure children have timely access to support to help them reach their potential, to provide information on prognosis and to allow families to gain support.
- A detailed history and clinical examination are key to diagnostic assessments.
- Cognitive assessment includes testing intellectual functioning and adaptive functioning.
- Genetic testing may be used to determine specific causes of IDD.

In the United Kingdom, children with suspected intellectual developmental disorder (IDD) (or global developmental delay [GDD] in those under 5 years of age) may first present in a number of different clinical settings. Parents, health visitors or nursery/school teachers may have concerns that prompt a referral to the GP. From here, children may end up being seen by a community paediatrician who specialises in children with developmental delay/neurodevelopmental disorders, or by a general paediatrician with a similar interest, a clinical geneticist or a child and adolescent psychiatrist. Many other professionals including doctors from other specialities may have been previously involved or may be involved in parallel, depending on when the child presented and what their other issues are (Box 11.1). There may also have been antenatal concerns (Box 11.2).

GDD is characterised by significant delay in two or more areas of developmental domains, including speech and language, fine and gross motor skills, cognitive abilities or activities of daily living. It is a diagnosis made in children under the age of 5. In some cases, the delay may be mild and transient. However, GDD can be predictive of a future diagnosis of IDD. It is important to be clear with families about whether a diagnosis of GDD made in early childhood should later be considered a diagnosis of IDD or not, because of the implications in terms of support available to the child and their family – some services may be specifically for people with IDD, but families may not realise that their child's diagnosis of GDD in early childhood would be considered IDD. Depending on their degree of ability, a child may or may not have had formalised cognitive testing and when this is not carried out there can be some difficulty in deciding whether a child (or later on, an adult) should be classified as having IDD.

Clinical assessment

The assessment of a child can encompass several different aspects and will typically involve determining (possibly at different times) whether they meet the criterion for IDD and ruling out/ruling in other differentials, investigating for underlying causes and assessing their functioning and the presence/absence of other comorbidities and medical/social issues (Figure 11.1). There can be a great deal of variation in this. It is important to remember that a child should be seen not just as an individual, but as a someone situated within a particular environment, which encompasses home, school, college or workplace. There may be particular needs according to their environment. Those with IDD/GDD can be among the most vulnerable members of society, often with similarly vulnerable parents/carers and siblings. Sometimes this may lead to concerns around neglect and a child/young person's welfare.

History

A detailed history from the parents or caregivers is a vital first step (see Figure 11.2). This often needs to be supplemented with information from clinical records and this becomes increasingly important with age, as memories fade, or with a looked-after or adopted child. In this situation adoptive parents may have received limited background information and it may be necessary to speak to social services. Sufficient time needs to be apportioned to obtaining this information and it is important to remember, given the genetic basis of these conditions, that parents may have their own difficulties with retaining information and communicating. The relevant areas that should be enquired about are detailed in Box 11.3.

ABC of Neurodevelopmental Disorders, First Edition. Edited by Munib Haroon.
© 2024 John Wiley & Sons Ltd. Published 2024 by John Wiley & Sons Ltd.

Box 11.1 **Professionals who might be involved in investigating a child with IDD/GDD**

- Health visitor
- GP
- Community paediatrician
- General paediatrician
- Child psychiatrist
- Neurologist
- Geneticist
- Neonatologist
- Speech and language therapist
- Physiotherapist
- Occupational therapist
- Dietician
- Clinical psychologist
- Educational psychologist

Box 11.2 **Antenatal screening and IDD**

In some countries, routine antenatal screening is used to assess the risk of particular conditions associated with IDD. In England, nuchal translucency measurement on ultrasound, combined with blood testing, is offered between 10 and 14 weeks' gestation to screen for:
- Down's syndrome (Trisomy 21)
- Edwards' syndrome (Trisomy 18)
- Patau's syndrome (Trisomy 13)

Patients may choose to be screened for one or more of these conditions, or may opt not to undergo screening.

When results indicate a higher risk of one of these conditions, further testing is offered, including amniocentesis and chorionic villus sampling. If these diagnostic tests confirm the presence of Down's, Edwards' or Patau's syndrome, pregnant people may face difficult decisions about whether to continue with their pregnancy or to have a termination.

Antenatal screening for these conditions is seen as controversial by some people, and it is important that parents have access to unbiased information on prognosis.

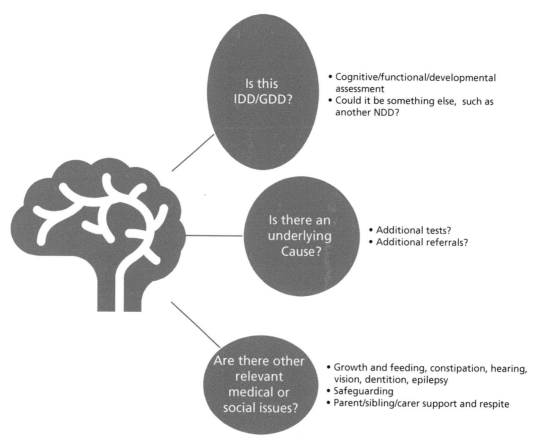

Figure 11.1 The assessment of a child/young person with intellectual developmental disorder (IDD)/global developmental delay (GDD) has a number of different aspects. NDD, neurodevelopmental disorder.

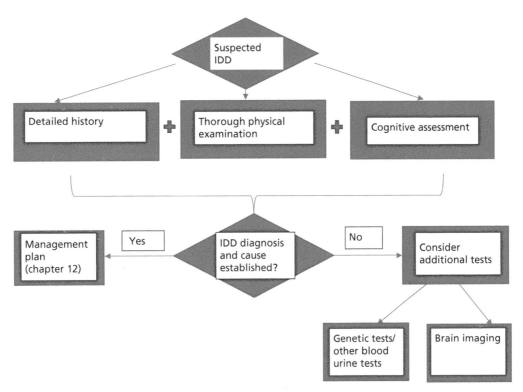

Figure 11.2 Steps in diagnostic assessment of a child/young person with possible intellectual developmental disorder (IDD). A degree of fluidity and pragmatism may need to be used in assessing a child based on commissioning arrangements and clinical presentation.

Examination

An examination of the child is the next important step. After the Covid-19 pandemic, in the era of the video consultation, it is worth thinking about what can be done via a video consultation and about the efficiency gains that may be obtained via such an approach, but also what essential elements may be lost.

A physical examination should be conducted carefully and sympathetically and tailored according to the child's individual needs and abilities. There is a lot to be said for adopting a 'hands-off' approach initially and gathering as much information as possible from observing the child's behaviour and appearance before laying hands on them. Similarly, communicating with the child is very important, not only because this is reassuring to them and makes them feel involved, but because it helps with arriving at a diagnosis. Children can offer unique insights into their situation and seeking this should not be neglected because of the assumption that children with IDD do not have something valuable to say. Clinicians may need to adapt their language, for example by using simple, short sentences, giving the child time to respond using whatever means of communication is effective for them. Caregivers should be encouraged to bring any resources to appointments that will aid in communication, such as photos or symbols, and clinicians should allow extra time for appointments.

A top-to-toe examination looking for symptoms and signs of an underlying disorder (Box 11.4) is important, but so is a developmental/cognitive assessment. Doctors do not always do formal cognitive testing in great depth, as it tends to be the domain of educational or clinical psychologists, although a number of standardised developmental tests address cognitive ability to some degree. Developmental assessments may be carried out by doctors according to the generally known milestones or through the use of a standardised tool (Schedule of Growing Skills, Griffiths 3). It is helpful, however, to remember that 'normality' in terms of achievement can be very variable. For example, while it is stated that children typically take their first steps at about 12 months of age, it is still considered to be within the normal range if a child does not do this until they are 18 months old.

Making a diagnosis of IDD can often require taking a pragmatic view of what is in the best interests of the child/young person and balancing this against the availability or lack of information and assessment tools. When such an approach is taken, it is worth documenting it in the records.

Cognitive and adaptive functioning assessment

Cognitive testing is used to evaluate the child's intellectual functioning compared to a typically developing child of the same chronological age. In the United Kingdom, the Weschler Intelligence Scale for Children (WISC) is commonly used and can give an indication of the child's overall intelligence quotient (IQ). Areas assessed include verbal comprehension, visuospatial skills, working memory, problem solving and reasoning. It is important that clinicians undertaking cognitive testing take into account any hearing or visual impairment.

Assessment of adaptive functioning is also needed to evaluate the child's ability to perform day-to-day activities, such as dressing themselves, feeding themselves and communication, compared to a typically developing child of the same age.

Clinicians interpreting these test results think carefully about whether any difficulties revealed by the tests can be explained by a learning disability. Multidisciplinary evaluation is often needed to exclude other causes of poor performance on cognitive and adaptive functioning tests, for example another neurodevelopmental disorder such as ADHD or autism spectrum disorder, or a language disorder.

Additional tests

There is a balance to be struck between over- and under-investigation. Tests can be invasive and unpleasant, and involve financial and time costs. Results may not be clear cut and false positives can necessitate additional unnecessary testing; however, failing to make a diagnosis could lead to a child or young person missing out on therapy or appropriate avenues of support and not having access to condition-specific information (such as on prognosis), or the family missing out on genetic counselling.

Which baseline tests are done will vary somewhat from one region to another and there is ongoing debate about what the best baseline investigations are; this will change over time as more refined genetic tests become cheaper and quicker. One possible set of baseline tests is shown in Box 11.5; further advice should be sought from local, regional or national guidance or from relevant clinicians. Testing should also be targeted according to the specific situation and be guided by clinical expertise. There may be little point in doing extensive investigations in a child with a clear history of pre-eclampsia or emergency caesarean who required resuscitation at birth, and who is not dysmorphic or showing other condition-specific features.

Blood:
- Full blood count
- Ferritin
- Urea and electrolytes
- Calcium
- Phosphate
- Liver function
- Alkaline phosphatase
- Urate
- Creatine kinase
- Amino acids
- Thyroid function
- Lactate
- Very long-chain fatty acids
- Acyl carnitine
- Transferrin isoforms

Urine:
- Organic acids
- Amino acids
- Glycosaminoglycans and oligosaccharides
- Sialic acid
- Sulfite

Genetics:
- Chromosomal microarray

Radiology
- Magnetic resonance imaging (MRI)

Table 11.1 Examples of specific genetic testing in intellectual developmental disorder with particular clinical features.

Syndrome	Clinical features	Specific genes affected
Fragile X syndrome	Long face Prominent forehead Large ears Macro-orchidism	*FMR1*
Cornelia de Lange syndrome	Short stature Thick eyebrows or synophrys (medial eyebrows meet in the midline) Short upturned nose Oligodactyly (absence of one or more fingers) Congenital diaphragmatic hernia Scoring systems based on clinical features are used to indicate whether or not genetic testing is indicated	*NIPBL, SMC1A, SMC3, RAD21, BRD4, HDAC8, ANKRD11*
Tuberous sclerosis	Ash leaf macules Adenoma sebaceum Shagreen patches Ungal/periungal fibromas Epilepsy Cardiac rhabdomyomas Benign kidney hamartomas Multiple pits in dental enamel	*TSC1, TSC2*
Coffin-Lowry syndrome	Short stature Downward-slanting palpebral fissures Flattened nasal bridge Short and tapering fingers Prominent forehead	*RSK2*
Rett syndrome	Normal development then hypotonia and loss of speech Purposeful hand use and stereotypical hand movements Gait abnormalities	*MECP2*

Less commonly, a child with GDD or IDD may have clinical features or a family history indicative of a specific disorder. In these cases, more specific genetic testing is helpful – although it is likely to be part of a panel of genetic tests (see Table 11.1 for examples).

The most useful genetic test at present is the chromosomal microarray, with reported diagnostic yields of 10–12%. There are issues with testing, including finding variants of uncertain significance (VOUS) that can be difficult to interpret, or incidental findings that are unrelated to the presentation and can lead to ethical implications – such as the finding of a gene that predisposes the carrier to dementia.

The range of genetic testing is opening up. It includes gene panel testing, whole-genome and exome sequencing, and may need to be considered in specific cases, for example in cases of unexplained GDD or IDD, especially where the presentation is at the moderate to profoundly severe end of the scale and a microarray was negative (see Chapter 30 for further details).

Referrals for whole-genome and exome sequencing are usually made by clinicians in paediatrics, neurology or clinical genetics. Ideally, the child and their biological mother and biological father should be tested, but when this is not possible, for example in children who have been adopted, single samples from the child themselves can be tested. As with chromosomal microarray, careful counselling of all those to be tested is needed due to the potential implications for the proband and their family. Families

undergoing testing may need support to understand issues around variable expression, and how environmental factors may affect the association between genotype and phenotype. As the understanding of genetic variants and their link with particular conditions continues to improve, the results and implications of genetic testing for individuals and their families may need to be re-evaluated over time. This means that individuals and their families, who may have been hoping that genetic testing would provide some certainty in terms of understanding the cause and prognosis of IDD, may have to live with a lengthy period of uncertainty.

The need for imaging studies also requires careful thought. Magnetic resonance imaging (MRI) can be very revealing, but it can feel claustrophobic, may require sedation or anaesthetic, and is not a cheap investigation. While some advocate a broad approach when it comes to investigating those with IDD, many advocate that MRIs are done in those with IDD who have accompanying micro/macrocephaly or abnormal neurological signs such abnormal tone, ataxia, optic atrophy or a seizure disorder.

It is important to exclude hearing difficulties and visual impairment for the purpose of differential diagnosis, but also because hearing and visual impairment occurs alongside IDD.

Conclusion

It may not be possible or necessary to decide on a complete approach to investigating a child at one visit, nor may it be within the field of one clinician to do so. Investigation and assessment can require a multidisciplinary approach. Having efficient networks for liaising with clinicians and other professionals can pay dividends in terms of achieving as close to an optimal approach as possible so that assessments can be done in a time-efficient manner.

Diagnosing IDD, any underlying cause and any comorbidities early is important to ensure that children receive timely access to support, treatment and interventions to optimise their potential and quality of life.

Further reading

American Psychiatric Association (2022). *Diagnostic and Statistical Manual of Mental Disorders*, 5e *Text Revision*. Washington, DC: American Psychiatric Association.

Mithyantha, R., Kneen, R., McCann, E. et al. (2017). Current evidence-based recommendations on investigating children with global developmental delay. *Archives of Disease in Childhood* 102: 1071–1076.

Vasudevan, P. and Suri, M. (2017). A clinical approach to developmental delay and intellectual disability. *Clinical Medicine* 17 (6): 558–561. https://doi.org/10.7861/clinmedicine.17-6-558.

CHAPTER 12

The Treatment of Intellectual Developmental Disorders in Children and Young People

Munib Haroon and Keri-Michèle Lodge

OVERVIEW

- As well as support for an intellectual developmental disorder, patients may require associated neurodevelopmental conditions to be treated alongside associated or incidental physical and mental health conditions.
- Assessing and treating conditions may be complicated by cognitive and/or communication difficulties.
- A change in behaviour may be the only sign that a child or young person is in pain.
- Special attention should be paid to avoiding inappropriate or over-medication, especially in children with multiple diagnoses.

While there is no treatment for intellectual developmental disorders (IDDs) themselves, different healthcare professionals are involved in many aspects of treatment and support (Figure 12.1). This includes providing professional guidance and support, where appropriate, on aspects of functioning and daily living and how to seek further support, understanding behaviours of concern, and identifying and treating underlying causes, managing/treating associated or underlying neurodevelopmental or mental health conditions and other associated or coincidental physical health conditions (Box 12.1).

The associated neurodevelopmental disorders (NDDs) include those mentioned throughout this book, such as autism and ADHD, while associated mental health conditions include anxiety and mood/depressive disorders. Common physical problems that may require treatment are outlined in Figure 12.2 and include sleeping difficulties, constipation and dental problems. But because of the range of conditions that may cause IDD, any system of the body may be involved. As such, this fact should always be kept at the forefront of a clinician's mind, and enquiring about conditions in a systematic fashion can help avoid something treatable from being missed.

As has been noted throughout this book, NDDs co-occur and so it is common for a child or younger person to require assessment and then treatment for one or more NDDs. The first challenge in this situation is often determining what conditions are actually present, because many features overlap and often one condition may mask another (see Box 12.2). It is not uncommon therefore for there to be some delay in having a clear picture of all the diagnoses that need to be managed and a child may go back and forth to a number of different clinics before a clear picture emerges. One way to try to limit such issues is to consider multiple diagnoses in one clinical setting. This is more likely to occur in a dedicated neurodevelopmental clinic with a single clinician assuming responsibility, as opposed to a child being seen in an ADHD clinic by one clinician and then in an IDD clinic by another. A further alternative, which may be more practical than redesigning the service, is to improve professionals' training and awareness about how such conditions co-occur so that they have a low threshold for arranging appropriate investigations.

Another challenge in diagnosing other clinical conditions is due to the communication differences and difficulties that individuals with IDD may have. It may be difficult for carers and healthcare providers to understand that a child or young person is in pain, and a change in behaviour may be the only sign of this (see Box 12.3). If a child with IDD is also autistic, which can sometimes be the case, then the presence of a high pain threshold or other sensory processing differences, such as delayed processing of pain, may compound this further. There is evidence, however, that professionals may sometimes assume that children and young people with IDD have a raised pain threshold even in instances when this is not true; this may subconsciously influence their assessment of pain, leading in some occasions to them administering less analgesia than is required.

Tackling the barriers to healthcare experienced by children and young people with IDD is a key aim of the NHS Long Term Plan (see Box 12.4). This includes rolling out the provision of annual health checks to all patients aged 14 years and above who are on the GP register of people with IDD (also referred to as the learning disability register) to meet unmet health needs that might otherwise be missed.

When children with IDD are treated for other neurodevelopmental conditions, it can become complicated for families and carers to understand the target of each treatment. Clarity is important for their understanding and to manage expectations. For example, if a

---

ABC of Neurodevelopmental Disorders, First Edition. Edited by Munib Haroon.
© 2024 John Wiley & Sons Ltd. Published 2024 by John Wiley & Sons Ltd.

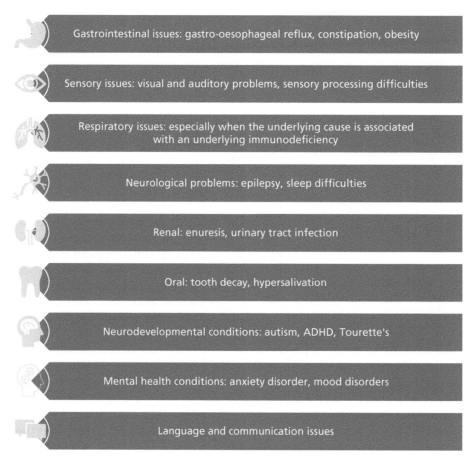

Figure 12.1 Health professionals may be involved in supporting a child with intellectual developmental disorder (IDD) in a number of different ways.

Gastrointestinal issues: gastro-oesophageal reflux, constipation, obesity

Sensory issues: visual and auditory problems, sensory processing difficulties

Respiratory issues: especially when the underlying cause is associated with an underlying immunodeficiency

Neurological problems: epilepsy, sleep difficulties

Renal: enuresis, urinary tract infection

Oral: tooth decay, hypersalivation

Neurodevelopmental conditions: autism, ADHD, Tourette's

Mental health conditions: anxiety disorder, mood disorders

Language and communication issues

Figure 12.2 A child with intellectual developmental disorder may require healthcare for a number of different conditions.

Box 12.1 **Leona**

Leona is 8 years of age. She was diagnosed with autism at the age of 3, and has recently been seen by an educational psychologist and a community paediatrician who has concluded (following a multidisciplinary assessment) that she has an IDD as well. She experiences disturbed sleep and is on melatonin to help regulate this. She has epilepsy, but her seizures are well controlled on sodium valproate. A month ago her sleep deteriorated and did not respond to a short-term increase in her melatonin. A check-up by her GP revealed that she had a tooth abscess. This responded well to antibiotics and her sleep is now back to where it had been.

Box 12.2 **Avoiding diagnostic overshadowing**

It is important to avoid diagnostic overshadowing, which occurs when clinicians incorrectly assume that the behaviour of a person with IDD is part of their IDD, rather than considering underlying causes, for example:
- Missed physical or mental health causes.
- Sensory impairments.
- Social issues, such as boredom, neglect or abuse.

child with IDD is also receiving treatment for ADHD because they are hyperactive, it is important to explain that methylphenidate may curb their hyperactivity, but may have a limited effect on other behavioural issues such as anxiety. Similarly, while treating inattention may help to improve some aspects of learning, there will still be limits on what may be achieved in a child with an underlying IDD.

A child with IDD and several associated conditions may be on a number of different medications. High dosages may be involved. It is important in every instance, but especially in more complex situations, to review each medication to think about whether it is the

Box 12.3 **Assessing pain**

Identifying pain in children and young people with IDD can be challenging. It helps to:
- Find out from the person themselves or their families/carers how they communicate in general. They may be more able to use pictures, symbols, signed language or assistive technology than spoken words.
- Ask the person themselves and their families/carers how they communicate pain.
- Consider whether they have a communication passport, which may include information on how they communicate pain.
- Take seriously what their families/carers tell you about whether they think the child/young person is experiencing pain.

Box 12.4 **Tackling the barriers to healthcare experienced by children and young people with IDD**

As part of the NHS Long Term Plan:
- NHS England and Improvement has provided guidance on identifying people with a learning disability/IDD so that accurate registers are kept
- Digital flags for IDD and autism will be implemented in electronic patient records.
- People with IDD aged 14 years and over are eligible for annual health checks.
- Children and young people with IDD in specialist residential schools are eligible for routine hearing, sight and dental checks.

Box 12.5 **Avoiding over-medication of children and young people with IDD**

NHS England has highlighted the need to avoid inappropriate medication in children and young people with IDD:
- STOMP (Stopping Over-Medication of People with a learning disability, autism or both) aims to reduce inappropriate use of psychotropic medication in children and young people with IDD and/or autism, and makes it clear that psychotropic medication should be seen as a last resort and, when prescribed, should be reviewed regularly.
- STAMP (Supporting Treatment and Appropriate Medication in Paediatrics) aims to ensure that children with IDD and/or autism and their families can access other treatment and support when children have behaviours that are difficult to manage, for example behavioural management support or other therapeutic support, and that when children do need medication they are able to access this, with regular reviews.

right medication for the situation, to consider drug interactions and to determine what the optimal dose is – is too much being given or too little? It is all too easy to continue prescribing a medication long after the signs are present that it is not working or that there are undesirable side effects (see Box 12.5).

A sometimes underappreciated function of the healthcare professional is to provide support, advice and reassurance to parents/carers and patients. This can take many forms and depending on the role may involve simple to increasingly complex behavioural advice and support, or signposting and referring to individuals who are better placed to provide this. This can often be accompanied with written material or recommending relevant websites and books, but there is a lot to be said for providing a personal touch. Often clinicians feels that the busyness of a clinic limits their abilities to perform this role and how this can be achieved is worth thinking about.

It is also important for clinicians to be aware of the limits of what they can advise and ask for. For example, while a paediatrician may be able to suggest what sort of interventions may help a child with IDD at school or what sort of school setting may be helpful, determining whether a child needs an Educational and Health Care plan (EHCP) or whether they should be educated in a mainstream or special school setting is ultimately a decision that will necessitate significant involvement from the local authority.

As with all aspects of healthcare, good record keeping is of great importance, so that parents have something to refer to and to share with relevant parties. This may include schools, especially when letters are not routinely sent to them, but also healthcare professionals. Families may apply for benefits and may request for a report from a healthcare professional, but often a clinical letter may suffice, and pertinent details on conditions and day-to-day functioning and activities of daily living can be extremely helpful, particularly when applications are rejected and matters end up in a tribunal.

Intellectual developmental disorders in hospitals

Children with an IDD are admitted to hospital more often than children without an IDD. They have higher rates of preventable mortality than the general population and experience poorer-quality care during hospitalisation. In 2015, NHS England launched the world's first national review of the deaths of people with IDD, the Confidential Inquiry into the deaths of people with learning disabilities, which aims to learn from avoidable deaths in this population and to reduce premature mortality. The more complex the needs of a child with IDD are, the more likely they are to experience adverse events. This can be addressed through training and knowledge, and, as part of the NHS Long Term Plan, a programme of mandatory training on learning disability and autism for those who work in both health and social care is being rolled out. The Equality Act 2010 also places a duty on those working in healthcare settings to make reasonable adjustments to ensure that health services are accessible to people with IDD (Boxes 12.6 and 12.7). All reasonable adjustments should be discussed with the child with IDD and their family, as the needs of each child with IDD will be unique. However, examples of such reasonable adjustments broadly include adapting communication to meet the needs of people with IDD, tailoring healthcare delivery and improving healthcare environments.

Box 12.6 **Making reasonable adjustments for children with IDD Using TEACH**

The TEACH mnemonic helps healthcare professionals remember key reasonable adjustments to consider for children with IDD:

T – Time: children with IDD will need longer to process information. Offering double or longer appointments as routine can help, and offering the first appointment of the day, when the waiting area is quieter and there is less chance of delay, can help manage their anxiety about having to come to an appointment.

E – Environment: consider which environment the child with IDD will be most comfortable in and where they will be most able to tolerate their encounter with the healthcare professional. This may mean offering home visits, for example for pre-operative assessments, or adjusting the environment, for example ensuring access to a quiet waiting area and staff covering up their uniforms if seeing these would provoke anxiety.

A – Attitude: every child should be treated with respect and dignity, and healthcare professionals should avoid making assumptions about a child with IDD's ability to engage in their consultation on the basis of their IDD. It is also important to view families/carers as experts by experience who can provide useful information to better understand the child with IDD.

C – Communication: healthcare professionals should adjust their communication to ensure it is accessible to the child with IDD, for example by using short sentences, avoiding jargon and explaining any new words. Some children with IDD may find pictures easier to understand than words. Others will have different ways of communicating, such as using Makaton signs, assistive technology or eye movements. Do not assume that a child with IDD who cannot speak is not able to understand.

H – Help: it is vital to harness the expertise of families/carers who know the child with IDD and can help healthcare professionals understand their child. It is also important to remember other sources of help, for example learning disability liaison nurses in hospital settings.

Box 12.7 **Karim**

Karim, 7 years old, is a boy with Down's syndrome, IDD, epilepsy and asthma. He was admitted to hospital with pneumonia, which also led to a deterioration in his seizure control. During his stay he experienced a prolonged seizure that was very distressing for his parents, but he made a full recovery and was discharged after a week in hospital. His parents wrote to the head of the department to offer their thanks and to suggest how his care and that of other children with IDD could be improved.

They felt that there should be systems in process for knowing that children about to be admitted had IDD. They suggested better training for staff so that they were more knowledgeable about IDD in general, but also Down's syndrome specifically, although they also wanted parents to be acknowledged as having special expertise when it came to their child. Specifically, they felt that some members of staff had not listened to their advice on managing Karim's episodes of challenging behaviour. They wanted staff not to make assumptions about pain control. They felt that Karim was under-administered analgesia because he was felt not to be showing obvious signs of pain, when in fact it was apparent to them from his behaviour that he was in considerable discomfort, and because of the belief that children with IDD had a lower sensation of pain. They felt that some staff were uncomfortable managing Karim and that there was an over-reliance on them (the parents) as a result.

They were nevertheless grateful for the staff's awareness of the importance of Karim's environment and their attempts to reduce excess noise and lighting by placing him in a cubicle and reduce over-stimulation during a ward round by having only one doctor enter the cubicle. They appreciated the use of photos to communicate, sensory resources and that the cubicle felt safe with bedrails. They offered to come and talk to the unit to help improve care for other children with IDD.

Transitions

Children with IDD and their families can experience significant barriers to accessing appropriate healthcare, as well as accessing the support they need in educational settings. Transitions can be particularly challenging because the support that the child and their family may have had to fight hard for can suddenly disappear. It can be an anxiety-provoking time, and families may not know which services can help once their child/young person reaches the age for being discharged from services for children and young people.

This is recognised in the NHS Long Term Plan, as part of which children and young people with IDD will be designated a key worker to help them navigate services during transition. Healthcare professionals also have an important role to play in supporting children and their families to cope with the challenges of transitions.

Further reading

Mimmo, L., Harrison, R., and Hinchcliff, R. Patient safety vulnerabilities for children with intellectual disability in hospital: a systematic review and narrative synthesis. *BMJ Paediatrics Open* 2 (1): e000201.

Oulton, K., Wray, J., Kenten, C. et al. (2022). Equal access to hospital care for children with learning disabilities and their families: a mixed-methods study. *Southampton: National Institute for Health and Care Research* https://doi.org/10.3310/NWKT5206.

Parkin, E. (2023). Learning disabilities: health policies. House of Commons Library. https://researchbriefings.files.parliament.uk/documents/SN07058/SN07058.pdf

CHAPTER 13

Intellectual Developmental Disorders in Adults

Keri-Michèle Lodge

> ### OVERVIEW
>
> - A diagnosis of intellectual developmental disorder (IDD) may be missed in childhood.
> - Adults with suspected IDD may present when the demands on them outweigh their abilities to cope, for example following the death of their family carer.
> - Adults with IDD experience significant health inequalities throughout their lifespan, including premature avoidable death, and annual health checks are an important way to detect unmet health needs.
> - When an adult with IDD presents with a change in behaviour, a biopsychosocial approach is essential to prevent diagnostic overshadowing and to avoid the inappropriate use of psychotropic medication.
> - The onset of dementia is often earlier in adults with IDD, particularly those with Down's syndrome.
> - At the end of life, adults with IDD and their carers should be involved in end-of-life and emergency care planning discussions.

Although intellectual developmental disorder (IDD) (or intellectual disability) is often diagnosed in childhood, for some people, particularly those with a milder intellectual disability, diagnosis may go unnoticed until adulthood. This chapter considers the specific challenges of diagnosing and managing IDD in adulthood.

Diagnosis of intellectual developmental disorder in adulthood

Like Alan in the vignette in Box 13.1, an individual's IDD can be missed until a change in their circumstances, for example difficulties at work or the death of an unpaid/family carer, brings them into contact with statutory services. In Alan's case, there are some features that may be suggestive of an IDD (see Box 13.2).

If there are several indicators of potential IDD, a formal intellectual disability diagnostic assessment should be considered. Undiagnosed IDD can result in low self-esteem and self-worth, or low mood, and can affect relationship and career choices. Although

there are potential benefits arising from having a formal intellectual disability diagnostic assessment (Box 13.3), being diagnosed with an IDD can result in feelings of shame and stigma. Adults with IDD are also vulnerable to harassment, exploitation and abuse.

A formal intellectual disability diagnostic assessment (Box 13.4) is a specialist task requiring the expertise of a multidisciplinary team. The aim is to exclude other potential causes of a person's difficulties, and to evaluate whether the individual meets the diagnostic criteria for IDD.

Management of intellectual developmental disorder in adulthood

The management of IDD in adulthood is diverse and depends on the individual's unique support needs. In general, although some adults with an IDD, particularly of mild severity, may live in the community without additional formal support, many will require support with education, employment and day-to-day care. Some, but not all, will require support from social care services, and some, but not all, will require support from specialist health services, such as community learning disability teams, where these are available.

Detecting unmet health needs and monitoring long-term conditions are important focuses of the management of IDD in primary care. It is important that those with an IDD are identified as such in their medical records, so that appropriate reasonable adjustments to care can be provided (Box 13.5). The person themselves, their families/carers or advocate, along with hospital learning disability liaison nurses, where available, can help identify reasonable adjustments required.

Any unpaid carers should be supported to identify themselves as such (rather than simply thinking of themselves as a person's parent or sibling, for example) and should be provided with information on sources of support for carers of people with an IDD. Carers/family members cannot make medical decisions on behalf of an adult with an IDD. In England and Wales, the principles of the Mental Capacity Act 2005 should be applied to adults with an IDD when making decisions about their healthcare and treatment (Box 13.6). The Mental Capacity Act is also relevant to other

ABC of Neurodevelopmental Disorders, First Edition. Edited by Munib Haroon.
© 2024 John Wiley & Sons Ltd. Published 2024 by John Wiley & Sons Ltd.

Box 13.1 **Alan**

Alan is a 20-year-old man who lives alone in a rented flat and works in an abattoir. He has a girlfriend, who rang the GP surgery to make an appointment for him. She got her mother to bring Alan to the surgery today because he did not know which bus to use. He was last seen by a GP at the age of 16 when he had broken a toe at the farm he had been working at, having left school with no qualifications.

Alan tells you, his GP, that he can't get to sleep at night. He has been late for work on some days and has been in trouble with his boss. Alan has been crying a lot. He tells you he got some letters in the post. His girlfriend read them to him because he cannot read. The letters were about unpaid bills. Alan does not know what to do. His girlfriend is cross with him because she wants him to give her some money so that they can get married. He does not have any contact with his family because, he says, his mother drinks and gets nasty, and his brother is currently in prison. He does not drink alcohol himself and has never used illicit drugs. You notice that he pauses before answering your questions and seems not to understand some of the words you use.

decisions, for example deciding whether to have sex or get married – this may be relevant in Alan's case (Box 13.1).

In a healthcare setting, the relevant clinician is responsible for assessing whether an adult with an IDD has the mental capacity to make the decision or not (Box 13.7) – for example, if the GP seeing Alan wishes to perform a blood test, they would first need to determine whether Alan had the mental capacity to consent to this.

A person may have the mental capacity to make some decisions but not others. For example, a woman with an intellectual disability and pain in her abdomen may be able to make a decision to consent to examination, but may lack the capacity to make a decision to consent to a hysteroscopy. It is therefore incorrect to make a blanket statement that a person lacks mental capacity to make medical decisions – mental capacity is both time and decision specific.

When a person is deemed to lack capacity, a best-interests decision is needed to decide which option is in the person's best interests, consulting with the person themselves as far as possible, their family and carers. Adults with an IDD may also have an independent mental capacity advocate to help ensure that the person's own values and preferences are taking into account. Some adults may also have a deputy for health and welfare – this is a person appointed by the Court of Protection to make certain

Box 13.2 **Features in history taking suggestive of an IDD in adults**

Medical history:
- Previous diagnosis of syndrome associated with intellectual disability, for example Down's syndrome
- Epilepsy
- Other physical disabilities or sensory impairments

Personal history:
- Pre-, peri- or post-natal environmental factors associated with the development of IDD, for example exposure to alcohol in utero, birth complications
- Family history of IDD or other neurodevelopmental disorder, although in previous generations this may not have been formally diagnosed and instead there may be a history of relatives attending 'special school' or living in institutions
- Delay in attaining childhood developmental milestones

Education:
- Attendance at 'special school'
- Difficulties with academic learning with poor academic attainment – may have left school early with no formal qualifications, or required extra help at school, such as one-to-one support in the classroom (in the United Kingdom, may have had a Statement of Special Educational Needs and/or an Education, Health and Care plan)
- Bullying due to poor academic attainment or seeming immature/being different to peers

Occupational history (paid and voluntary):
- Difficulties learning new skills or understanding and remembering new information at work, which may have led to getting into trouble with managers
- Unemployment

Relationship history:
- Difficulties understanding social cues
- May have a history of being exploited by peers, for example having their money taken by others

Day-to-day living skills:
- Difficulties with communication
- Difficulties in eating and drinking, staying warm and appropriately clothed, keeping clean (need for assistance with these tasks may be subtle)
- Difficulties using transport independently
- Difficulties with managing money, for example working out the change from £5.00 if buying a loaf of bread for £1.20

Box 13.3 **Benefits of a diagnostic assessment**

Benefits of an intellectual disability diagnostic assessment in adulthood:
- Answering questions about lifelong and current difficulties
- Opportunity for support, for example reasonable adjustments at work and when accessing healthcare or social care support
- Opportunity for annual health checks and health action plans

Box 13.4 **Components of an intellectual disability diagnostic assessment**

- In-depth history taking with the individual themselves, and with a carer/family member/friend who knows them well
- Review of school reports and childhood medical records
- Mental state examination
- Physical examination for features suggestive of a potential cause of IDD, for example syndromes with particular phenotypic features
- Investigations may include genetic testing – the approach to this varies globally and is dependent on local resources; brain imaging may also be undertaken
- Assessment of intelligence, for example using standardised, culturally appropriate intelligence quotient (IQ) tests, taking into account any additional sensory impairments such as visual or hearing impairment
- Assessment of functional skills, for example using standardised assessments of abilities in day-to-day life skills, such as preparing a hot drink

Box 13.5 **Reasonable adjustments for people with IDD**

Under the Equality Act 2010, there is a legal responsibility to ensure that public services, including health and social care, are accessible to people with a disability, including an IDD. This can be achieved by making reasonable adjustments, for example:
- Providing written information in an accessible format, for example using an 'easy read' approach or symbols, simple language and short sentences
- Allowing extra time
- Offering the first or last appointment of the day when the environment is less busy
- Providing a quiet waiting area
- Allowing carers to accompany the person to their appointment if appropriate
- Allowing carers to stay with the person throughout an admission to hospital
- Allowing the person to visit the hospital prior to a planned admission or procedure to provide an opportunity for desensitisation or coordinating care so that multiple procedures, for example blood tests, dental examination, ophthalmic examination, can be carried out under one period of sedation/anaesthesia

Box 13.6 **Mental capacity and decision making**

In England and Wales, the Mental Capacity Act 2005 states that every adult, regardless of whether they have an IDD or not, has a right to make their own decisions wherever possible. The five main principles of the Act are:
- Assume that the person is able to make a decision.
- Do everything practicable to support the person to make the decision themselves, for example providing information in an accessible format.
- Do not assume that a person lacks the mental capacity to make a decision because you think their decision is unwise.
- If a person is found to lack the mental capacity to make a decision themselves, the decision made must be in the person's best interests.
- Any decisions, treatment or care for someone who lacks mental capacity must be the option least restrictive of their human rights and freedoms.

Box 13.7 **Assessing mental capacity**

The Mental Capacity Act 2005 sets out a two-stage test of mental capacity:
- Does the person have an impairment of their mind or brain (for example, arising from an IDD)?
- Does the impairment mean the person is unable to make the specific decision when they need to?

A person is deemed to lack the mental capacity to make the specific decision at the time they need to if they are unable to:
- Understand the information relevant to the decision – the person should be provided with accessible information and be given time and support to understand this
- Retain that information
- Use or weigh that information as part of decision making
- Communicate their decision (this can be by any means, for example an adult with an IDD with communication difficulties may use signs or eye movements rather than speech)

Physical health

People with an IDD have a higher prevalence of particular physical health problems compared to the general population (see Box 13.8), but the barriers to accessing healthcare faced by people with intellectual disability result in missed or delayed diagnosis and treatment.

Detecting physical health conditions can be challenging in people with an IDD who have difficulties making themselves understood to others, and whose presentation may be atypical – a change in behaviour may be the only indicator of an underlying health condition.

People with an IDD die at a younger age than people in the general population (see Figure 13.1), with 6 out of 10 dying before the age of 65, compared to 1 in 10 of the general population in 2021. According to a report into the avoidable deaths of people with IDD (White et al. 2022), 49% of all deaths of people with an IDD were

decisions on behalf of an adult who lacks mental capacity to make them themselves. When agreement on what would be in the person's best interests cannot be reached, the decision may have to go before the Court of Protection.

Box 13.8 **Common physical health comorbidities seen in adults with IDD**

- Epilepsy
- Mobility difficulties
- Sensory impairment, for example undetected visual impairment
- Dysphagia
- Gastro-oesophageal reflux disease
- Poor oral health
- Constipation
- Obesity

Box 13.9 **Factors contributing to the premature avoidable deaths of people with an IDD**

- Lack of reasonable adjustments, e.g. failure to provide information in an accessible format
- Lack of investigations in the community when families/carers/advocates highlighted concerns
- Poor information sharing between primary and secondary care
- Poor understanding and application of the Mental Capacity Act 2005
- Poor involvement of people with an IDD and their families/carers/advocates in 'do not attempt cardiopulmonary resuscitation' decisions

Source: Data from White et al. (2022).

avoidable, compared to 22% in the general population. People with an IDD who also have epilepsy or are from a Black, Asian or minority ethnic background are also particularly likely to die at a younger age. Institutional discrimination is one of the key factors in the premature avoidable deaths of people with an IDD (Box 13.9).

In the United Kingdom, annual health checks play an important role in identifying unmet health needs in people with an IDD (see Box 13.10). Assumptions should not be made about the person's lifestyle – they may be sexually active, may drink alcohol and might smoke or use recreational drugs.

Adults with an IDD should be provided with accessible information on public health screening, including cervical screening tests, breast screening and self-examination, and testicular self-examination. As people with an IDD age, they may require support to access regular dental checks, hearing checks, sight tests and podiatry.

Box 13.10 **Annual health checks**

People aged 14 and over who have moderate, severe or profound IDD, or people with a mild IDD and other complex health needs such as autism, are entitled to an annual health check in primary care.

Annual health checks:
- Identify undetected health conditions early
- Evaluate the appropriateness of ongoing treatments
- Promote health, e.g. screening and immunisation

Mental health

Adults with an IDD may have other comorbid neurodevelopmental conditions, such as autism. Estimates of the prevalence of mental health conditions in adults with an IDD vary; however, research suggests there are higher rates of conditions such as depression among adults with an IDD compared to adults in the general population. The reasons for this are complex and include differences in brain architecture and differential exposures to psychosocial determinants of mental ill-health, such as poverty and social exclusion.

Assessing the mental health of adults with an IDD can be challenging due to communication barriers and atypical presentation (see Box 13.11), for example a change in behaviour. It is important to

Box 13.11 **Presentation of mental health difficulties in adults with IDD**

- Change in behaviour, for example increased vocalisations
- Loss of interest in activities they usually enjoy
- Social withdrawal and avoidance
- Irritability
- Agitation
- Increased/decreased need for sleep
- Loss of usual skills, or increased need for prompting with day-to-day life skills

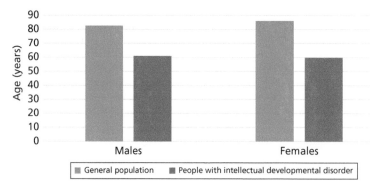

Figure 13.1 Median age of death in people with an intellectual developmental disorder compared to the general population. *Source:* Data from White et al. (2022).

speak to the person with an intellectual disability first (see Box 13.12), but talking to a family member or carer who has known the person well for a long time is also essential. Transitions can be particularly challenging for adults with an intellectual disability and can be a key trigger to changes in behaviour.

In England and Wales, specialist community learning disability teams, composed of psychiatrists specialising in intellectual disability psychiatry, psychologists, learning disability nurses, speech and language therapists and occupational therapists, provide specialist mental health assessment and support to people with an IDD and a health need, such as a mental health need, which cannot be met by 'mainstream' services.

When an adult with an IDD presents with a change in behaviour, there is a risk that this change may be attributed to the individual's IDD rather than considering the possibility of an underlying physical or mental health cause – this is diagnostic overshadowing (see Chapter 12). To avoid this, a biopsychosocial approach should be taken to differential diagnosis (see Box 13.13).

Sometimes an adult with IDD may engage in 'behaviour which challenges', also known as 'challenging behaviour' (Box 13.14). This is not a diagnosis and the underlying cause of the behaviour should be elucidated (see Box 13.13).

Once any underlying causes have been identified and addressed, analysis of the behaviour, its triggers and its consequences is needed so that those supporting the individual can modify the triggers and consequences to diminish occurrence of the behaviour – this is known as a behaviour management plan.

There are no licensed pharmacological treatments for behaviour which challenges in adults with IDD. However, when psychosocial interventions, such as a behaviour management plan, are ineffective,

Box 13.12 **Clinical tip**

Adults with an IDD are vulnerable to abuse, which can be perpetrated by carers, friends or family members who accompany the person to their medical appointments. It is important to speak to the person with an IDD alone.

Box 13.13 **Underlying causes to consider in adults with an IDD presenting with a change in behaviour**

Biological factors:
- Pain, including dental pain, or ingrown or infected toenails
- Gastrointestinal problems, particularly constipation, gastro-oesophageal reflux
- Infection, for example of ears, urinary tract, respiratory tract, skin
- Sensory impairments, for example visual loss (e.g. cataracts), hearing loss (e.g. wax occlusion)
- Medication side effects

Psychological factors:
- Mental health problems, e.g. depression

Social factors:
- Social or environmental stressors, e.g. loss of carer/relative/peer, abuse, neglect, boredom

Box 13.14 **Behaviour which challenges**

Behaviour of such intensity, frequency or duration that it threatens the physical safety of the person or others, or restricts their access to community facilities, for example:
- Physical aggression to self, e.g. biting or hitting self
- Physical aggression to others, e.g. hitting, kicking, biting others
- Damaging the environment or property, e.g. throwing and breaking objects

or when the behaviour is associated with severe risks to the individual or to others, psychotropic medication can be considered to target specific symptoms, for example a selective serotonin reuptake inhibitor (SSRI) to reduce anxiety.

People with an IDD are at risk of inappropriate use of psychotropic medication, and NHS England has made the STOMP (stopping over medication of people with a learning disability, autism or both) pledge to tackle this.

Where possible, mental health difficulties in adults with an IDD should be assessed and treated in the community. If a person is at risk of admission to a mental health hospital (known in England and Wales as an Assessment and Treatment Unit), it is important that those involved in the person's health and social care convene to determine how best to manage the situation with the aim of ensuring that hospital admission is a last resort.

Ageing with an intellectual developmental disorder

As adults with an IDD age, they experience similar challenges to those without an IDD, for example regarding their sexuality, and they should be provided with accessible information on understanding sex and relationships. Adults with an IDD are vulnerable to sexual abuse and exploitation, and where there are concerns about this, the local adult safeguarding team should be engaged.

Some adults with an IDD may become parents, and may require additional support to cope with the demands of pregnancy, childbirth and parenthood.

For adults with an IDD who live with their parent carers, the ageing and death of their parents can be particularly difficult to cope with. Accessible bereavement and trauma support may be needed.

Dementia and intellectual developmental disorders

Although the overall prevalence of dementia in people with IDD is comparable to that of the general population, prevalence is higher in adults with Down's syndrome, at around 56% in those aged 60 and over. Age of onset of dementia is earlier in people with an IDD, although diagnosis can be difficult due to atypical presentation (see Box 13.15).

It is recommended that every adult with Down's syndrome should have a baseline dementia assessment by the age of 30 years, which can be used as a comparison in the future should changes in the person's cognitive or adaptive functioning be suspected.

Box 13.15 **Features of dementia in IDD**

- Memory loss may be less obvious
- Progressive loss of previous self-care skills may be an earlier feature
- Carers may report a generalised 'slowing down'
- Progressive dysphagia and choking are seen in the early stages of dementia in people with Down's syndrome
- Development of epilepsy is prominent in dementia in people with Down's syndrome

---

Regular cognitive screening of adults with Down's syndrome aged 40 years and over should be considered as part of health action planning.

Diagnosis of dementia in intellectual developmental disorder

As with any change in behaviour, when an adult with an IDD presents with a suspected decline in their cognitive functioning, a broad differential diagnosis is needed (see Box 13.16).

Screening for the factors in Box 13.16 can be undertaken in primary care, with onward referral to secondary care for a full dementia diagnostic assessment where this is indicated. This may require the use of diagnostic assessment instruments specifically tailored to people with an IDD.

Management of dementia in intellectual developmental disorder

Current research suggests that it is difficult to draw conclusions about the effectiveness of pharmacological interventions in dementia in adults with an IDD.

Ensuring that the person's carers have had specific training on dementia is vital.

Box 13.16 **Differential diagnosis of dementia in IDD**

Sensory impairments:
- Hearing
- Vision

Physical health issues:
- Hypothyroidism
- Vitamin B_{12} deficiency
- Obstructive sleep apnoea
- Side effects of prescribed medications

Mental health difficulties:
- Depression

Environmental factors:
- Change or loss of family, friends or usual carers, peers
- Change of accommodation, e.g. moving to a new room or home
- Lack of stimulation or boredom
- Abuse

Death and dying with intellectual developmental disorder

Adults with an IDD and their families, carers or advocates should be involved in discussions about 'do not attempt cardiopulmonary resuscitation' decisions and around emergency healthcare planning. An IDD should not be deemed a reason to withhold care and treatment at the end of life, and should not, in itself, be recorded as a cause of death on a person's death certificate.

In England and Wales, all deaths of people with an IDD aged 4 years and over (along with those of autistic people aged 18 and over) are investigated by a national mortality review project (known as LeDeR; White et al. 2022), with the aim of learning from areas of both good and poor practice to prevent future avoidable premature deaths.

Further reading

British Psychological Society (2015). Guidance on the assessment and diagnosis of intellectual disabilities in adulthood. https://www.bps.org.uk/guideline/guidance-assessment-and-diagnosis-intellectual-disabilities-adulthood

British Psychological Society and Royal College of Psychiatrists (2015). Dementia and people with learning disabilities. https://www.bps.org.uk/guideline/dementia-and-people-intellectual-disabilities

Equality Act 2010. https://www.legislation.gov.uk/ukpga/2010/15/pdfs/ukpga_20100015_en.pdf

Heslop, P., Blair, P.S., Fleming, P. et al. (2014). The confidential inquiry into premature deaths of people with intellectual disabilities in the UK: a population-based study. *Lancet* 383 (9920): 889–895.

Mental Capacity Act. 2005. https://www.legislation.gov.uk/ukpga/2005/9/pdfs/ukpga_20050009_en.pdf

National Institute for Health and Care Excellence (NICE) (2015). Challenging behaviour and learning disabilities: prevention and interventions for people with learning disabilities whose behaviour challenges [NICE guideline NG11]. https://www.nice.org.uk/guidance/ng11

National Institute for Health and Care Excellence (NICE) (2016). Mental health problems in people with learning disabilities: prevention, assessment and management. NICE guideline [NG54]. https://www.nice.org.uk/guidance/ng54

National Institute for Health and Care Excellence (NICE) (2018). Care and support of people growing older with learning disabilities. NICE guideline [NG96]. https://www.nice.org.uk/guidance/ng96

NHS England (2017). Stopping Over-Medication of People with a learning disability, autism or both (STOMP): toolkit for reducing inappropriate psychotropic drugs in general practice and hospitals https://www.england.nhs.uk/wp-content/uploads/2017/07/stomp-gp-prescribing-v17.pdf

White, A., Sheehan, R., Ding, J. et al. (2022). *Learning from Lives and Deaths – People with A Learning Disability and Autistic people (LeDeR) Report for 2021*. London: Autism and Learning Disability Partnership, King's College https://www.kcl.ac.uk/ioppn/assets/fans-dept/leder-main-report-hyperlinked.pdf

CHAPTER 14

An Introduction to Tic Disorders and Tourette's Disorder

Fraser Scott

OVERVIEW

- Tics are common in childhood, especially in boys, and may start from 2 years of age.
- Tourette's disorder has an estimated prevalence in children and adolescents of 0.7% and is a primary movement disorder.
- Tics can be motor or vocal and although initially involuntary, often patients develop a premonitory urge beforehand that can help them to block or delay the tic occurring.
- Comorbidities, e.g. attention deficit hyperactivity disorder, obsessive compulsive disorder or autism, are commonly seen in patients with Tourette's.

History

The first published case report of tics was in 1825 by French doctor Jean-Marc-Gaspard Itard. In 1885, Georges Gilles de la Tourette published a case series of nine patients ('Maladies des tics') and his mentor, Jean–Martin Charcot, later recommended the newly recognised condition be named after his pupil (Tourette's disorder or Tourette's syndrome). It was regarded as a psychiatric disorder until the twentieth century, when the neurological basis for the condition was recognised because of a favourable response to neuroleptics.

Definitions and features

The key features of a tic are that it is a sudden, recurrent, rapid, non-rhythmic and involuntary movement, affecting either skeletal (motor) or laryngeal (vocal) muscles. Neurophysiological studies have confirmed the involuntary nature of these movements by documenting a lack of preceding *Bereichtschaftspotential*. This term is German for 'readiness potential' and is an electrical discharge measured in the motor cortex and supplementary motor area before a voluntary movement.

In distinction to other movement disorders, although tics often will first manifest as truly involuntary, over time the patient will become aware of a warning (premonitory urge) that precedes the tics. These sensory phenomena will often cause a feeling of internal distress that is temporarily relieved by allowing the tics to happen.

Tics can be motor or vocal (verbal) and simple or complex. Common examples are shown in Table 14.1.

Over time the patient will build up a repertoire of tics. The tics will wax and wane and may change from one type to another. Most movements are sudden and involve quick contractions of muscles or groups of muscles, although dystonic or tonic contractions can also be seen.

The tics will be more likely to be seen when the patient is stressed, tired, or unwell and will diminish when they are asleep. They often will flare up at the end of the school day when the child comes home or when they are relaxing watching TV. Tics are frequent and sudden and can occur with little warning, so minor injuries can occur as well as muscle pain from repetitive, strenuous contractions.

A patient with Tourette's (or other tic disorder) is often suggestible, so just discussing tics in clinic may trigger the occurrence of a bout. In addition, some tics may be consistently triggered by external stimuli. Over time a patient may learn how to temporarily control or suppress their tics.

Usually, a patient will start with simple motor tics, with more complex movements and vocal tics developing later (on average one to two years after the appearance of the motor tics). Often the motor tics will start in the face, neck and shoulders and may then progress over time to affect other regions of the body. A patient may develop a cluster of associated complex tics, often linked with disinhibited behaviour. Attention deficit hyperactivity disorder (ADHD) can be present from an early age, although obsessive compulsive disorder (OCD)-related behaviours like touching or tapping tend to develop later.

A compulsive element to tics can develop where patients will feel a need to even things up or make things feel right. In addition, self-injurious behaviour can develop, often in association with complex motor tics, which are more commonly seen in patients who also have ADHD and rage attacks.

Table 14.1 Examples of motor and vocal tics.

	Simple	Complex
Motor	Eye blinking	Touching things
	Shoulder shrugging	Combination of movements
	Screwing up nose	Gestures
		Copropraxia
		Dystonic or tonic tics
Vocal	Sniffing	Shouting out
	Coughing	Coprolalia (uttering obscene or
	Throat clearing	inappropriate remarks/words)
	Noises	Echolalia (repeating heard speech)
		Palilalia (repeating one's own speech)

Classification

The classification is similar between DSM-5-TR and ICD-11.

Tic disorders commence before the age of 18 and are not attributable to any other disorder (e.g. Huntington's disease) or medication. It is very unusual for them to begin after this age and when this occurs there is usually some other identifiable disorder or explanation, or a careful enquiry will reveal a subtle history of tics during childhood. Depending on the chronicity/persistence and the presence of vocal or motor tics, or both, they will generally be classified as Tourette's disorder, persistent (chronic) motor or vocal tic disorders or a provisional tic disorder. In Tourette's disorder, there are multiple motor and one or more vocal tics present – although not all at the same time – which may wax and wane but will have persisted for over a year. In persistent motor or vocal tic disorders, the key difference is that there is not a mix of motor or vocal tics, but only tics in one category (there may be

several types of motor or vocal tics). A provisional tic disorder has been present for less than one year and so can eventually, with persistence, shift into one of the other two categories (Figure 14.1).

Epidemiology

Tics are common in childhood, and even Tourette's disorder, once thought of as a rare entity, is now increasingly recognised in 0.3–1% of the population. In the largest study from Denmark, the incidence was 9.1 per 1000. In most children tics will be 'primary', although they can occur secondary to acquired brain injury, genetic or metabolic disorders or as a side effect of medications. There is commonly a family history of either tics, OCD or ADHD.

Tics are commoner in boys than girls, with a ratio of 3–4 : 1, and often start around the age of 5 years, although they can start younger. Usually, the condition is worst when the child finishes junior school and begins high school (8–12 years) and in the majority it has completely or significantly settled by the time the patient turns 18, although symptoms can persist and even worsen into adulthood.

Comorbidities

A patient with Tourette's disorder may have their tics as the sole manifestation of the condition but more commonly, as seen in Figure 14.2, they have associated difficulties. These comorbid conditions can be more problematic then the tics themselves and can predate the onset of tics or manifest later in childhood. Table 14.2 lists some of the commoner problems seen in these patients.

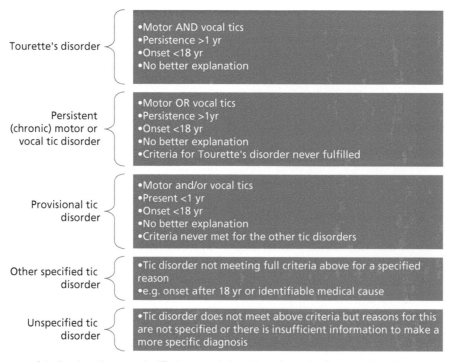

Figure 14.1 The different types of tic disorders. These mostly differ in terms of chronicity and the mix of motor and vocal tics.

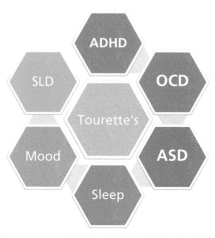

Figure 14.2 Common comorbidities in Tourette's disorder: ADHD, attention deficit hyperactivity disorder; ASD, autism spectrum disorder; OCD, obsessive compulsive disorder; SLD, specific learning difficulty. Sleep and mood related problems are also very common.

Often the patient may have several of these problems, which can be entangled in a negative feedback loop.

Learning difficulties are common, which is not surprising given the list of accompanying comorbidities, although the intelligence quotient (IQ) of patients with Tourette's syndrome is typically within the normal distribution.

Quality of life is therefore adversely affected by having Tourette's. There is a functional impairment with social repercussions and there is also an impact on family functioning, as well as a higher psychiatric morbidity in carers and family.

Pathophysiology

There has been considerable progress in understanding the mechanisms behind tics and Tourette's, although a full unified theory is still eluding researchers.

The cortico-striatal-thalamo-cortical (CSTS) circuits seem key to understanding both the tic movements themselves as well as the premonitory urges that precede them and the commonly associated OCD and ADHD behaviours. Various areas within the cortex seem relevant to the spectrum of Tourette's, including not just the pre-motor and supplementary motor areas but also the emotional centres in the limbic system, as well as cognitive centres in the frontal lobe. These areas connect to numerous sites in the basal ganglia, thalamus as well as cerebellum and finally project back to the cortex. Structural magnetic resonance imaging (MRI) scans have shown abnormal cortical thickness levels in the areas described, while functional MRI scans have shown abnormal connections within the described network.

Virtually all the neurotransmitters are involved in the areas described, including dopamine, glutamate, GABA, serotonin, acetylcholine, histamine, noradrenaline, endogenous cannabinoids (CB1 and CB2 receptors), adenosine and opioids. This may explain why a wide range of medications with different mechanisms of action have shown efficacy in ameliorating tic severity. Unfortunately, it is also the reason why no single agent has shown superiority in tic management.

Genetics plays a significant role. This was suggested by Tourette himself, and most practitioners will be accustomed to recognising the increased frequency of tics, OCD, ADHD and so on in the families of their patients. There is no single gene identified that causes these disorders, but rather a mix of common and rare alleles that

Table 14.2 Comorbidities in Tourette's.

Comorbid condition	Estimated % in patients with Tourette's	Additional information
ADHD	60	
Sleep problems	60	
OCD	30	
ASD	20	
Mood problems	30	Anxiety
		Depression
		'Rage attacks'
Self-injurious behaviour	30	Linked not just to tic severity but to OCD, rage attacks and impulsivity
Externalising behaviours	14	Conduct disorder
		Oppositional defiant disorder
Other neurodevelopmental difficulties and issues	10	Dyspraxia
	Common	Specific learning difficulty
	Common, especially with ADHD	Executive function difficulties
Sensory processing difficulties	80 (self-report from Tourette's syndrome patients)	Sensitive to sensations, which may lead to either excessive avoidance or seeking behaviours
Other medical conditions with increased prevalence		Migraine
		Epilepsy
		Restless legs syndrome
		Asthma, allergy and other atopic conditions

ADHD, attention deficit hyperactivity disorder; ASD, autism spectrum disorder; OCD, obsessive compulsive disorder.

confer different degrees of risk and explain some of the variations in the severity of presentation. This is not surprising given the complex circuitry involved. Epigenetics and environmental triggers are also thought to be a crucial factor influencing time and manner of presentation.

Inflammation, included that related to infection, seems to be a factor in some patients, with a temporal link between acute infections and the appearance of tics. Streptococcal infection is best described, and the specific condition of PANDAS (paediatric autoimmune neuropsychiatric disorder associated with streptococcal infection) is described in the next section. Other infectious agents have also been described, including mycoplasma pneumoniae, chlamydia pneumoniae/trachomatis, toxoplasma gondii, enteroviruses and others. Other evidence for an immune hypothesis includes altered cytokines or autoantibody levels in Tourette's patients, as well as a response to either antibiotics or immunomodulatory therapies, including steroids, intravenous immunoglobulin or plasmapheresis. There is also an increased incidence of asthma, coeliac disease and autoimmune thyroid disease.

It is theorised that the patient may inherit an abnormal stress response that affects the hypothalamic–pituitary–adrenal axis as well as limbic and autonomic systems. Molecular mimicry may then allow abnormal antibodies (generated in response to an intercurrent infection) to target sites in the CSTC circuit, leading to the various manifestations of tic disorders. Environmental factors may also influence age of onset indirectly through epigenetic effects. Finally, there is increasing recognition of the role that the gut as a distinct nervous system plays in its interaction with the central nervous system as well as of the influence of the gut microbiome on neurological symptoms, including Tourette's syndrome.

PANDAS

This clinical entity was first described in 1998, when an association was recognised between movement disorders (principally tics, or choreiform movements), OCD and streptococcal infection.

More recently, in 2012, a related condition, PANS (paediatric acute-onset neuropsychiatric syndrome) was also identified.

The latest proposed diagnostic criteria are shown in Table 14.3, although at the time of writing these have not been classified within ICD-11 or DSM-5-TR.

There are now both American and UK clinician guidelines related to diagnosis, investigation and treatment, although a recent publication could find no statistical association between streptococcal infection and tic exacerbations.

The conditions have proven controversial, as was summarised in a consensus statement from the British Paediatric Neurology Association (BPNA), released in 2021. The main issue was around lack of randomised controlled trial (RCT) data to support a guideline as well as concern about the use of antibiotics, non-steroidal anti-inflammatory drugs, steroids and other more invasive immunomodulatory therapies, and again the lack of significant, consistent evidence to justify treatments with potentially serious side effects. Recommendations from the BPNA included a multidisciplinary approach involving paediatric neurology and mental health, among others; consideration of the wide differential for these symptoms;

Table 14.3 Summary of diagnostic criteria for PANDAS and PANS.

PANDAS	PANS
Presence of OCD ± tics (often multiple, complex or unusual)	Abrupt, acute dramatic onset of OCD or severely restricted food intake
Age of onset between 3 years and puberty	No age requirement
Acute onset and relapsing/remitting course	Not better explained by a known neurological or medical condition
Association with group A streptococcal infection	Severe, acute and concurrent symptoms from at least two of the following categories:
Association with neurological abnormalities (motor hyperactivity or choreiform movements)	Anxiety
	Emotional lability/depression
	Irritability, aggression, severe oppositional behaviour
	Behavioural (developmental) regression
	Deterioration in school performance
	Motor or sensory symptoms
	Somatic symptoms/signs: sleep disturbance, enuresis or urinary frequency

OCD, obsessive compulsive disorder; PANDAS, paediatric autoimmune neuropsychiatric disorder associated with streptococcal infection; PANS, paediatric acute-onset neuropsychiatric syndrome.

and caution about prescribing antibiotics, steroids or other immunomodulatory therapies. Further research is clearly needed as well as collaboration with patients, their families, charities and other professional organisations.

Further reading

British Paediatric Neurology Association (BPNA) (2021). Consensus statement on childhood neuropsychiatric presentations, with a focus on PANDAS/PANS. https://bpna.org.uk/?page=pans-pandas

Chowdhury, U. and Murphy, T. (2017). *Tic Disorders: A Guide for Parents and Professionals*. London: Jessica Kingsley Publishers.

Dalsgaard, S., Thorsteinsson, E., Trabjerg, B.B. et al. (2020). Incidence rates and cumulative incidences of the full spectrum of diagnosed mental disorders in childhood and adolescence. *JAMA Psychiatry* 77 (2): 155–164.

Forde, N.J., Kanaan, A.S., Widomska, J. et al. (2016). TS – EUROTRAIN: a European wide investigation and training network on the etiology and pathophysiology of Gilles de la Tourette syndrome. *Frontiers in Neuroscience* 10: 1–9.

Freeman, R. (2015). *Tics and Tourette Syndrome: Key Clinical Perspectives*. London: Mac Keith Press.

Geng, J., Liu, C., Xu, J. et al. (2022). Potential relationship between Tourette syndrome and gut microbiome. *Jornal de Pediatrica* 14: 1–6.

Girgis, J., Martino, D., and Pringsheim, T. (2022). Influence of sex on tic severity and psychiatric comorbidity profile in patients with pediatric tic disorder. *Developmental Medicine & Child Neurology* 64: 488–494.

Isaacs, D. and Riordan, H. (2020). Sensory hypersensitivity in Tourette syndrome: a review. *Brain & Development* 42 (9): 627–638.

Jafari, F., Abbasi, P., Rahmati, M. et al. (2022). Systematic review and meta-analysis of Tourette syndrome prevalence; 1986–2022. *Pediatric Neurology* 137: 6–16.

Martino, D. and Leckman, J. (2022). *Tourette Syndrome*, 2e. Oxford: Oxford University Press.

Martino, D., Schrag, A., Anastasiou, Z. et al. (2021). Association of group A Streptococcus exposure and exacerbations of chronic tic disorders. *Neurology* 96: e1680–e1693.

Openneer, T.J.C., Forde, N.J., Akkermans, S.E.A. et al. (2020). Executive function in children with Tourette syndrome and attention-deficit/hyperactivity disorder: cross-disorder or unique impairments? *Cortex* 124: 176–187.

Rae, C.L., Critchley, H.D., and Seth, A.K. (2019). A Bayesian account of the sensory motor interactions underlying symptoms of Tourette syndrome. *Frontiers in Psychiatry* 10: 1–15.

Singer, H., Mink, J., Gilbert, D., and Jankovic, J. (2021). *Movement Disorders in Childhood*, 3e. New York: Academic Press.

Swedo, S.E., Leckman, J.F., and Rose, N.R. (2012). From research subgroup to clinical syndrome: modifying the PANDAS criteria to describe PANS (pediatric acute-onset neuropsychiatric syndrome). *Pediatric and Therapeutics* 2 (2): 1–8.

Swedo, S.E., Leonard, H.L., Garvey, M. et al. (1998). Pediatric autoimmune neuropsychiatric disorders associated with streptococcal infections: clinical description of the first fifty cases. *American Journal of Psychiatry* 155 (2): 264–271.

Tourette Association of America (n.d.). Understanding behavioral symptoms in Tourette syndrome: TS is more than tics. https://tourette.org/resource/understanding-behavioral-symptoms-tourette-syndrome/#:~:text=TOURETTE%20SYNDROME%20BEHAVIORAL%20SYMPTOMS%201%201.%20DYSINHIBITION%20Difficulty,FLIGHT%E2%80%99%20…%208%208.%20DIFFICULTIES%20WITH%20TRANSITIONS%20

Ueda, K. and Black, K.J. (2021). A comprehensive review of tic disorders in children. *Journal of Clinical Medicine* 10: 1–32.

CHAPTER 15

The Assessment and Diagnosis of Tic Disorders

Fraser Scott

OVERVIEW

- Diagnosis requires history taking, examination and review of abnormal movements, either in clinic or by reviewing video footage.
- Tourette's is a primary diagnosis, so usually no further investigations are required.
- There are a variety of validated scales for assessing tic severity.
- Functional tics have become more widely recognised.

Initial assessment

The starting point for a child or young person referred with abnormal movements is a detailed history and examination.

Useful details to explore during the history (as well as a description of the movement itself) are shown in Table 15.1.

When assessing children with movement disorders, age of onset and therefore suspected aetiology are key considerations that will dictate further investigations (magnetic resonance imaging [MRI], metabolic work-up, genetics, etc.). Identification of other associated problems (learning problems, upper motor neuron signs, deficits in vision or hearing, epilepsy, etc.) is also important, as this may allow recognition of specific clinical syndromes.

Detailed family neurological history is important as specific genes (e.g. *CACNA1A*, *PRRT2*) can be inherited in families but cause a variation in age and type of clinical presentation, for instance familial hemiplegic migraine (FHM), ataxia or developmental and epileptic encephalopathy (DEE).

Children and young people with tics may well have active tics during the consultation, either spontaneously or after the variety of movements has been discussed, as often patients are suggestible. Families should be encouraged to catch a variety of video clips showing different movements at home using smartphones/tablets if they are not witnessed in clinic.

General and neurological examination should be performed, including assessing height, weight and head circumference as well as checking blood pressure and looking for evidence of neurocutaneous stigmata, assessing speech, gait and eye movements as well as upper and lower limb neurology. Other abnormal movements may be seen during history taking or examination, and simple manoeuvres can be used to assess for tremor, myoclonus, choreoathetosis or dystonia. Examination is typically normal in those with a primary tic disorder such as Tourette's. Some of the features that can help differentiate tics from stereotypies and myoclonus are detailed in Table 15.2.

From this detailed clinical assessment, a range of abnormal movements can be differentiated (Figure 15.1).

Tics/Tourette's disorder is a clinical diagnosis and is usually a *primary* condition, hence further investigations are not usually required.

Further assessment

Assessment of severity and impact of the tics can be quantified with a variety of clinical scales, the best known of which is the Yale Global Tic Severity Scale (YGTSS). This rates motor and phonic tics based on current levels as well as worst ever, and looks at different criteria including number, frequency, intensity, complexity and level of interference with voluntary activity. There is also a final score for level of impairment caused by the tics, giving a total score between 0 and 100. The scale can be found online (https://pandasnetwork. org/wp-content/uploads/2018/11/YGTSS.pdf) and is free to download and use.

The validity of a clinical diagnosis of Tourette's syndrome can be measured using the Tourette Syndrome Diagnostic Confidence Index. This correlates well with YGTSS, although it should be noted that certain clinical features like complex tics or copro-phenomena, which are weighted in favour of the diagnosis, are not likely to be present when the patient is younger. (Copro-phenomena are obscene words or gestures.)

A screening tool like the Strengths and Difficulties Questionnaire (SDQ) can also be helpful. Again, this can be found online (https://www.sdqinfo.org/a0.html), where questionnaires and manual scoring can be downloaded for free. There is online electronic scoring of SDQ (https://sdqscore.org/SDQ), which requires an administrator account to be set up. There is a cost for each patient's questionnaire scoring ($0.25 in 2022). Hopefully it

---

ABC of Neurodevelopmental Disorders, First Edition. Edited by Munib Haroon.
© 2024 John Wiley & Sons Ltd. Published 2024 by John Wiley & Sons Ltd.

Table 15.1 Relevant factors to explore from history taking.

Background details from history	Specific details about movement
PMH including birth	Age of onset
Medication; illicit substance use	Body distribution
FH – movement disorders, OCD, ADHD, ASD	Temporal patterns
	Effect on QoL and education
Development and learning history	Aura or premonitory feeling before
Emotional issues/mental health	Exacerbating/relieving factors

ADHD, attention deficit hyperactivity disorder; ASD, autism spectrum disorder; PMH, previous medical history; FH, family history; OCD, obsessive compulsive disorder; QoL, quality of life.

will be soon available for free across NHS England, although individual trusts may need to set up accounts.

There are various questionnaires assessing quality of life (QoL) in children with chronic conditions including some developed specifically for children and young people with Tourette's.

The premonitory urge (which children come to recognise as an unpleasant sensation preceding the tic and can be temporarily relieved by doing the tic) can also be rated using the Premonitory Urge for Tics Scale (PUTS).

Where the history has suggested the presence of comorbidities such as attention deficit hyperactivity disorder (ADHD), obsessive compulsive disorder (OCD) or autism spectrum disorder (ASD), then relevant screening tools are available – Swanson, Nolan and Pelham (SNAP) scale, Connors, Yale Brown Obsessive-Compulsive Scale (Y-BOCS) and so on – and onward referral to the appropriate team for detailed assessment would be indicated.

Educational or neuropsychology assessment may be helpful – certainly, it is important to assess whether there are learning difficulties and the extent to which the tics are having impacts on school life. Executive dysfunction is more common in Tourette's syndrome, with effects on both planning and emotional regulation. There are various tools that can be used to assess this, the most widely used of which is Behavior Rating Inventory of Executive Function (BRIEF).

Emotional health and resilience should be considered. There are screening tools for depression and anxiety – Beck Depression Inventory (BDI), Hospital Anxiety and Depression Scale (HADS) and so on – and a referral to Child and Adolescent Mental Health Services (CAMHS) is often beneficial, as will be discussed in Chapter 16.

Usually, tics and Tourette's are a primary (presumed genetic) disorder, although rarely tics can occur secondary to an underlying neurological disorder, usually because of damage or genetic/metabolic conditions. These include:

- Infections: encephalitis, Lyme's disease, human immunodeficiency virus (HIV)
- Cerebral damage: stroke, head trauma, poisoning (carbon monoxide, mercury)
- Genetic conditions: Fragile X, Retts, neurocutaneous disorders
- Neurodegenerative disease: neuro-acanthocytosis, Huntington's, dentatorubral-pallidoluysian atrophy (DRPLA), neurodegeneration with brain iron accumulation (NBIA)
- Systemic illness: Behcet disease

In addition, medications or illicit substances can also cause tics, including:

- L-Dopa or neuroleptics
- Antiepileptics, e.g. lamotrigine, carbamazepine, phenytoin
- ADHD treatments, e.g. Ritalin®
- Amphetamines, cocaine, ecstasy

Tics can also occur as one form of a *functional* movement disorder (FMD).

Table 15.2 Stereotypies with different hyperkinetic movements seen in children.

	Motor stereotypies	Tics	Myoclonus
Age of onset	Under 3 yr	4–8yr	Any age
Pattern	Remains constant; parents may be able to predict	Variable; progress in rostro-caudal (top-to-toe) direction	Usually constant
Movements	Flapping or dyskinetic movements of hands and arms, trunk; head nodding	Variable: patient builds up repertoire that will wax and wane	
Noises	Humming	Variable: simple noises or words/phrases	Gasp or shout: forced exhalation from diaphragm
Precipitant	Excitement, tiredness, being engrossed, anger	Stress, anxiety, excitement	Tiredness
Duration	Can last several minutes	Short, can be repetitive	Individually very short; can occur in clusters
Premonitory urge	No	Yes	No
Distraction	Yes	Temporary	No
Suppressibility	Yes	Yes	No
Family history	Sometimes	Often (tics or comorbidities)	Sometimes if epileptic
EEG	Normal	Normal	Abnormal if epileptic
Associated problems	ASD; LD	ADHD; OCD; ASD	Epilepsy
Natural history	Can persist, especially if complex or associated with ASD/LD	Two-thirds will settle or improve over time	Variable depending on underlying cause

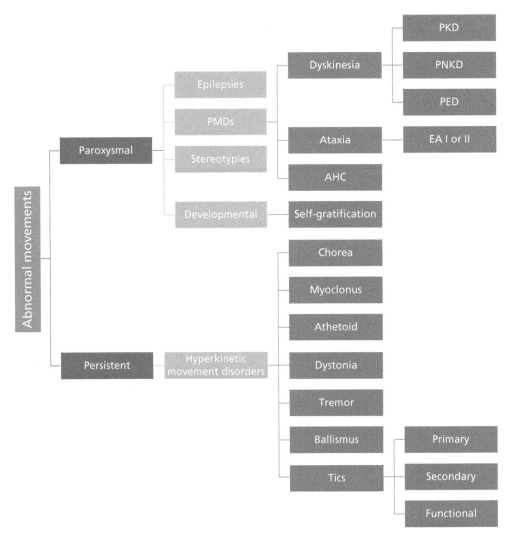

Figure 15.1 Abnormal movements in children. AHC, alternating hemiplegia of childhood; EA, episodic ataxia; PED, paroxysmal exercise-induced dyskinesia; PKD, paroxysmal kinesiogenic dyskinesia; PMD, paroxysmal movement disorder; PNKD, paroxysmal non-kinesiogenic dyskinesia.

Functional movement disorders

Initially described in adults, where they are a common diagnosis for patients referred to a neurology or movement disorder clinic, FMDs are being increasingly recognised in children. In older children and teenagers, as in adults, they are commoner in females, although the sex ratio is more equal for younger children. Functional MRI scans have shown abnormal signalling between networks involving the prefrontal cortex, limbic regions and basal ganglia, confirming a demonstrable, physical substrate for this functional problem.

The diagnosis rests on the clinical assessment of history and examination, supplemented by reviewing video footage of typical attacks. Other somatic symptoms are more commonly seen as well as other functional neurological disorders (FNDs) such as dissociative (non-epileptic) seizures. Some clues to the diagnosis are listed in Table 15.3, although this is not an exhaustive list. 'La belle indifference' is literally translated as beautiful ignorance, in the face of an apparent serious illness. Entrainment relates to when the

Table 15.3 Relevant details to explore from history and examination of a patient with a suspected functional neurological disorder.

History	Examination
Abrupt and severe onset	Inconsistency
Link to recent injury or illness	Distractibility
Precipitated by recent psychological stressor	Entrainment
	Signs not consistent with
Variability	neuroanatomy
'La belle indifference'	Specific clinical signs, e.g. Hoover's sign

frequency of a motor sign in a limb switches to match the frequency of tapping carried out by another limb.

Using a more traditional psychological approach, predisposing, precipitating and perpetuating factors can often be identified.

Long-term prognosis is better in children and young people compared to adults, although the key to a successful outcome rests with the patient and family accepting and understanding the functional diagnosis as well as appropriate psychological management and support. A multidisciplinary team approach is often essential to link social care, education and physical rehabilitation with psychology and neurological input.

There are several online resources and support for FND, including FND Guide (www.neurosymptoms.org). This has an additional online 'formulation tool' that allows patients or families to summarise their symptoms as well as the degree to which each is affecting daily life. The tool summarises all the inputted information into a PDF report that can be shared with health or education professionals.

Functional tic-like behaviours

Functional tics have traditionally been recognised as a rare subtype of FMDs. The numbers seen, however, have increased dramatically in the last few years. This is thought in part to be a consequence of the global Covid-19 pandemic, which altered children's and young people's normal routine, causing feelings of uncertainty and fear as well as social isolation. The other factor thought to be responsible for the increased numbers of children and young people presenting with functional tics is the influence of social media, especially video-sharing platforms like YouTube and TikTok.

Like the paradigm seen in epilepsy patients (where alongside their typical epileptic seizures they can later develop non-epileptic or dissociative seizures), some patients with functional tic-like behaviours (FTLBs) may have had more typical tics when younger (up to 40% in some publications). More commonly patients develop their FTLB rapidly (sometimes overnight) with no preceding history, in their teenage years, and females are significantly over-represented. Usually there is no increased incidence of the typical comorbidities seen in typical tics (like ASD or ADHD).

Some may have other functional symptoms, and there may be an obvious trigger like anxiety or trauma. There is a higher incidence of anxiety or depression. These children and young people are more likely to have presented at the emergency department and have a higher level of self-injury and aggression. They are more likely to have prolonged 'tic-like attacks' with abnormal regulation of movements, often accompanied by symptoms resembling those of anxiety or panic attacks.

Their motor tics may look similar, although they are less likely to involve the head and face and often have a less stereotyped nature. The tics are more complex, and copropraxia (obscene or inappropriate gestures) is more frequently seen. There is an increased prevalence of coprolalia and other complex vocal tics. The FTLBs are suggestible (like typical tics) but also are distractible.

These children and young people often lack the premonitory urge commonly described in similarly aged typical tic patients and struggle to suppress their tics. The typical waxing-and-waning natural

history is frequently missing and the FTLBs more commonly affect normal activities, especially those the patient perceives as unpleasant. As a result, attendance at school is disproportionately affected compared to typical Tourette's.

Management is similar to the approach used for other FNDs: clear explanation of the nature of the condition, a multidisciplinary approach and involvement of clinical or neuropsychological support. Maintaining normal routines and maximising healthy eating, sleeping and exercise habits can be helpful. Identifying and reducing reinforcement, either positive or negative, is also important. These patients will not usually respond to anti-tic medications.

There is a functional tic leaflet available on the FND Guide website: https://www.neurosymptoms.org/en_GB/symptoms/fnd-symptoms/functional-tics

Further reading

Brandsma, R., Van Egmond, M.E., and Tijssen, M.A.J. (2021). Diagnostic approach to paediatric movement disorders: a clinical practice guide. *Developmental Medicine & Child Neurology* 63: 252–258.

Eapen, V. and Usherwood, T. (2022). Assessing tics in children. *BMJ* 376: 1–5.

Han, V.X., Kozlowska, K., Kothur, K. et al. (2022). Rapid onset functional tic like behaviours in children and adolescents during COVID-19: clinical features, assessment, and biopsychosocial treatment approach. *Journal of Paediatrics and Child Health* 58: 1181–1187.

Horner, O., Hedderly, T., and Malik, O. (2022). The changing landscape of childhood tic disorders following COVID-19. *Paediatric and Child Health* 32 (10): 363–367.

Larsh, T., Wilson, J., Mackenzie, K.M. et al. (2022). Diagnosis and initial treatment of functional movement disorders in children. *Seminars in Pediatric Neurology* 41: 1–12.

Leckman, J.F., Riddle, M.A., Hardin, M.T. et al. (1989). The Yale global tic severity scale: initial testing of a clinician-rated scale of tic severity. *Journal of the American Academy of Child and Adolescent Psychiatry* 28 (4): 566–573.

Openneer, T.J.C., Tarnok, Z., Bognar, E. et al. (2020). The premonitory urge for tics scale in a large sample of children and adolescents: psychometric properties in a developmental context. An EMTICS study. *European Child and Adolescent Psychiatry* 29: 1411–1424.

Robertson, M.M., Banerjee, S., Kurlan, R. et al. (1999). The Tourette syndrome diagnostic confidence index: development and clinical associations. *Neurology* 53 (9): 2108–2112.

Silveira-Moriyama, L., Kovac, S., Kurian, M.A. et al. (2018). Phenotypes, genotypes, and management of paroxysmal movement disorders. *Developmental Medicine and Child Neurology* 60: 559–565.

Su, M.T., McFarlane, F., Cavanna, A.E. et al. (2017). The English version of the Gilles de la Tourette – quality of life scale for children and adolescents: a validation study in the United Kingdom. *Journal of Child Neurology* 32 (1): 76–83.

Woods, D.W., Piacentini, J., Himle, M.B., and Chang, S. (2005). Premonitory urge for tics scale (PUTS): initial psychometric results and examination of the premonitory urge phenomenon in youths with tic disorders. *Developmental and Behavioural Pediatrics* 26 (6): 397–403.

CHAPTER 16

The Management and Outcome of Tic Disorders

Fraser Scott

OVERVIEW

- All children with tic disorders should receive adequate explanation and support – this is called psychoeducation.
- There should be a consistent approach both at home and at school, recognising aggravating or reinforcing factors.
- Management of comorbidities may be more important than tic suppression.
- Psychological support is key.
- Medication is reserved for a small number of patients whose tics are detrimental to their physical, mental, social or educational health.

This chapter describes the different treatment modalities available to help patients with chronic tic disorders such as Tourette's disorder. Figure 16.1 summarises a step-wise, pragmatic approach, based on evidence supporting use of different interventions.

Psychoeducation and support

Management of children and young people with a chronic tic disorder starts with explaining the diagnosis to them and their family. The discussion is around the nature of the condition, commonly associated problems and ways in which family and school can support the patient.

Involvement of school/college is essential so that their approach to the child or young person and their tics will be non-judgmental and non-punitive. Emotional as well as learning support is key and all those involved with the patient should adopt a similar approach.

This provision of information and holistic support is termed *psychoeducation* and is essential to all those newly diagnosed. In some patients, this may be all that is required to allow them to live with their condition without it causing a negative impact until the expected spontaneous improvement later in the teenage years. Often it can be helpful to consider aggravating and relieving factors/situations as well as unintended reinforcing elements that may occur because of the tics.

Supporting and developing self-esteem and resilience are important and often there can be a beneficial effect from developing extracurricular activities and hobbies – particularly sport or music.

There are charities supporting people with tics and Tourette's. The website for the UK charity Tourettes Action (www.tourettes-action.org.uk) has a lot of useful information for patients, families, clinicians and teachers. It also has downloadable patient-held documents, including a Tourette's syndrome 'passport' and information on tic attacks. Canada and the United States have their own charities and the Canadian Child & Parent Resource Institute has useful information: https://www.leakybrakes.ca/brake-shop/brake-shop-virtual-clinic.

Treat comorbidities, sleep and pain management

As previously mentioned, comorbidities should be identified and managed appropriately. This may reduce stress levels for the child or young person, which may in turn reduce exacerbation of the tics. Also, certain medications used to treat certain comorbidities – like attention deficit hyperactivity disorder (ADHD) or obsessive compulsive disorder (OCD) – may also have a secondary benefit of reducing tics, which may be the case for clonidine and guanfacine (Box 16.1).

Sleep problems are common and will exacerbate not just tics but also mood and learning problems. Assessment in a sleep clinic, looking at the sleep schedule, and sometimes short courses of medication like melatonin, can have a beneficial effect.

Forceful motor tics can cause physical pain from repetitive or violent muscle contractions. The pain can in turn worsen the tics, as well as causing functional impairment to the patient. Chronic pain from any cause has long been recognised as affecting mental health, and this is certainly seen in patients with long-standing tics, who have lower quality-of-life scores and higher rates of depression. In their most extreme form, the tics can cause injuries or physical damage: 'malignant' tics. Management should address not only the pain itself but also the psychosocial impact. Support is therefore needed as well as analgesia, distraction and relaxation techniques. Self-help techniques including massage, stretching, and hot or cold packs can be helpful.

ABC of Neurodevelopmental Disorders, First Edition. Edited by Munib Haroon.

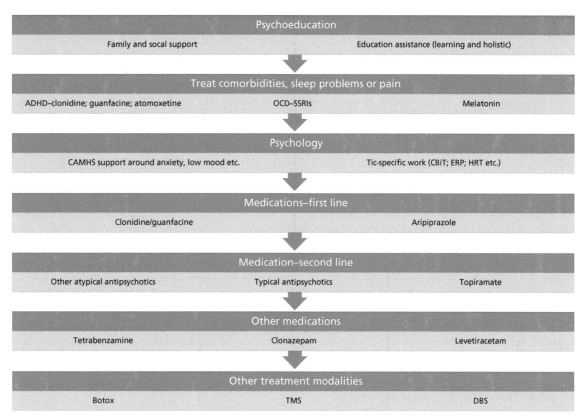

Figure 16.1 Summary of management approach. ADHD, attention deficit hyperactivity disorder; CAMHS, Child and Adolescent Mental Health Services; CBiT, comprehensive behavioural intervention for tics; DBS, deep brain stimulation; ERP, exposure and response prevention; HRT, habit reversal training; OCD, obsessive compulsive disorder; SSRI, selective serotonin reuptake inhibitor; TMS, transcranial magnetic stimulation.

Box 16.1 Treating ADHD or OCD with co-occurring tic disorder

Tic disorders and ADHD

Standard ADHD medications such as methylphenidate can still be used in patients who also have tics or a formal diagnosis of Tourette's, and this is clearly stated in the National Institute for Health and Care Excellence (NICE) guidelines on ADHD management. Rarely, a patient taking stimulants may develop tics. It may be that this is a drug side effect, in which case benefits of treatment should be weighed against problems caused by the tics. There should be a discussion with family about reducing dose or changing to alternative ADHD medication. Alternatively, the occurrence of tics maybe a coincidence and related to the waxing and waning, natural temporal pattern of tics and Tourette's. The alpha-adrenergic agonists (clonidine and guanfacine) can be used for this co-presentation. There is some published evidence showing benefit of these medications in treating tics.

Tic disorders and OCD

There is a NICE guideline, updated in 2019, on management of OCD and it is beyond the scope of this chapter to review this in detail. Guidance from the European Society for the Study of Tourette Syndrome notes that children with Tourette's respond as well to selective serotonin reuptake inhibitors (SSRIs) as those without it, and that the same can be said for cognitive behavioural interventions. The same guidance, however, cites evidence from other trials stating that higher doses may be required, along with the attendant increased risk of side effects. In treatment-resistant cases, while neuroleptics may be added alongside SSRIs, there is a limited evidence base and a need for drug safety monitoring. There is an increased risk of neuroleptic malignant syndrome (NMS) in those taking both neuroleptics and SSRIs.

Psychology

Referral to Child and Adolescent Mental Health Services (CAMHS) is often the next step in management. It can provide support around general mood problems such as anxiety, depression, anger or self-harm. There are several online self-help support sites for mental health problems from a variety of providers, including www.kooth.com and www.youngminds.org.uk.

Once these sessions have been completed, more specific focused work on the tics can start, with either comprehensive behavioural intervention for tics (CBiT) or exposure and response prevention (ERP).

CBiT includes a combination of psychoeducation and habit reversal training plus other aspects such as relaxation training, as well as helping to develop an understanding of the context surrounding the tics. This will include the situations that may trigger or worsen the tics as well as the unintended consequences of tics (both positive and negative) that will reinforce the tic cycle. Once a patient has found an urge and accompanying tic, work can focus on developing a competing response or tic blocker. This is an active movement that will prevent the tic from occurring. It should be easy and unobtrusive for the patient to perform. Length of treatment is usually in weekly sessions of 8–10-week blocks. The patient and family are expected to practise the techniques at home and will often have a workbook to complete and keep track of progress.

Both CBiT and ERP are evidence-based and effective treatments, although they require the child or young person to have awareness of their premonitory urge that goes with the tic, so often are reserved for older children. They look to address internal or external triggers to reduce the frequency and severity of tics and therefore minimise their impact. There is compelling evidence to support the efficacy of these forms of behavioural therapy, which of course avoid side effects from medications. Traditionally delivered face to face, there is growing evidence that they are still effective when delivered virtually – something that became necessary during the Covid-19 pandemic.

Finally, cognitive behavioural therapy is available and can be helpful, again for older patients.

First-line pharmacological management

Medication for tics is often reserved for when psychological options have been tried unsuccessfully or where there is objective evidence of harm because of the tics. This harm may be physical (pain or injury), psychological, social or educational.

There are currently no NICE guidelines for management of tics and Tourette's, but there are evidence-based guidelines from both the American Academy of Neurology and the European Society for the Study of Tourette Syndrome.

All medication should be prescribed by those with appropriate experience according to relevant national guidance/formularies.

Guanfacine
The efficacy of different medications (at best 30% reduction in tics) must be balanced against their potential side effects. Guanfacine (typically Intuniv, modified release) has a long half-life, meaning it is generally well tolerated with fewer side effects compared to clonidine and can also be given once a day. Medication is generally commenced at 1 mg (in those over 6 years of age and 25 kg in weight) and titrated on a weekly basis in accordance with the British National Formulary (BNF). It can take a few weeks for the effects to become noticeable and this needs to be explained to the child or young person and their parents/carers. Medication needs to be titrated carefully, and ongoing monitoring of growth parameters and blood pressure/pulse is required. There is a risk of hypotension while on the drug and also hypertension, especially after abrupt withdrawal, which should be avoided.

Clonidine
General paediatricians maybe more familiar with clonidine, which also has evidence of modest benefit in tic management and is usually well tolerated with a lack of significant side effects for most patients. Clonidine is available as 25 µg and 100 µg tablets. There is also a 50 µg/5 ml sugar-free liquid preparation and a transdermal patch. It should be used with caution in depression, bradyarrhythmia, constipation and heart failure.

General advice is to start with 1.5–3 µg/kg/d, divided in 2–3 doses. Depending on the weight of the patient and their ability to swallow tablets, it is usually easiest to start with 25 µg, beginning with a night-time dose and increasing to twice or three times daily. Total daily dose can be increased every 3–5 days, although a slower build-up improves tolerability and allows the family to judge the efficacy at reducing the number and severity of tics. It is generally well tolerated. Common side effects include tiredness, dizziness (especially postural) or dry mouth.

The maintenance dose for tics is 3–5 µg/kg/d with a maximum of 300 µg/d.

Baseline blood pressure and monitoring as the dose increases should be performed and if weaning off, then a slow reduction is recommended to avoid rebound hypertension.

Atomoxetine
Atomoxetine is a pre-synaptic selective norepinephrine reuptake blocker, which is an effective ADHD treatment that can be trialled if standard stimulants are not tolerated. There is less evidence showing its benefit in treating tic disorders compared to clonidine/guanfacine.

Second-line medications

Antipsychotics
Balancing evidence of benefit with a favourable side-effect profile, the atypical antipsychotic aripiprazole is typically trialled first. Risperidone, quetiapine and olanzapine have also been used. Often a lower dose is used than with schizophrenia, which helps with tolerability.

Older typical antipsychotics such as haloperidol, pimozide or sulpiride have also been used. There is limited evidence for these and an increased risk of side effects.

These medications need close supervision and monitoring. Each neuroleptic has specific side effects (including drowsiness, cognitive effects, obesity and electrocardiogram [ECG] changes). Depending on the mode of action, some may have antimuscarinic side effects or may elevate prolactin, causing gynaecomastia or even galactorrhoea. Less common but more concerning are the extrapyramidal side effects (including akathisia, parkinsonism or tardive dyskinesia). Although rare, there is also the risk of NMS.

Anti-epileptics
Topiramate, clonazepam and levetiracetam are the commonest anti-epileptic drugs used for management of tic disorders. Topiramate has the most published evidence and both American and European guidelines suggest its use in treatment-resistant cases.

Other medications

There is currently no compelling evidence supporting the use of vesicular monoamine transporter type 2 inhibitors, such as tetra-benazine, or dopamine antagonists, such as metoclopramide.

Other treatment modalities

Botulinum toxin ('Botox') has been used to treat persistent tics, localised to a specific area, although this has been tried only in older adolescents and adults.

Another option is non-invasive brain magnetic stimulation, such as repetitive transcranial magnetic stimulation (rTMS), which generates a magnetic field that passes through the skull and can affect cortical excitability, assessed by measuring motor evoked potentials. This can be delivered either continuously or intermittently, often through theta burst stimulation. Another method is transcranial direct current stimulation (tDCS). This is less well established but has the potential benefits of being cheaper and easier to administer. These treatments target areas closer to the surface such as the supplementary motor area and primary motor cortex, as the basal ganglia would be too deep for the superficial currents to reach.

Surgery in the form of deep brain stimulation has been shown to be helpful for the minority of patients with severe tics who have not responded to psychological and pharmacological treatments. Due to the areas targeted, it can also help with OCD symptoms. It is available in only a few specialised centres.

There is anecdotal evidence showing benefit of cannabidiol (CbD) in adults. Formulations with a higher concentration of tetrahydrocannabinol (THC) seem more likely to be helpful, although they are also more likely to cause side effects. Currently in the United Kingdom, the licence to prescribe medicinal CbD (Epidyolex) is restricted to the treatment of specific genetic epilepsies in tertiary neurology centres.

There is no convincing published data supporting the use of dietary supplements such as magnesium, zinc, B-complex vitamins and omega-3 fatty acids, although there are anecdotal accounts of individual improvements.

Prognosis, outcome and adult care

Outcome is traditionally divided into thirds, where one-third find that their tics resolve over time; a second group have persistent tics, which are not as severe as during childhood/adolescence and often find that OCD becomes their main issue; and a final third continue to have persistent and problematic tics (Figure 16.2). Recent research suggests that a worse outcome is more likely in female

patients. A small proportion of patients have persistently severe or worsening tics as adults.

Many patients with persisting mild tics learn to accommodate them into their daily life and may develop hobbies or even pursue careers that require focused attention, as this can minimise tic severity – examples include sports, playing musical instruments and brick laying. Predictors of long-term tics may include number and severity of complex tics and a strong family history of tics. Comorbid ADHD or OCD can be associated with psychosocial dysfunction in adulthood, but it is hard to untangle whether this is a direct effect of those comorbidities or a consequence of persisting tics.

There is a higher proportion of functional tics in adult patients and (as has been mentioned earlier) they can coexist in patients who also have Tourette's.

Medications used to treat tics (which are limited in their efficacy and can cause significant side effects) will not work for functional tics. A biopsychosocial model should be adopted to understand the presenting symptoms and management should be directed to psychology/psychiatry.

There is a link between Tourette's and other chronic health problems, including diabetes, autoimmune conditions and heart disease, which can lead to morbidity and affect quality of life.

There is excess mortality compared to the standardised mortality ratio for the general adult population. Some of this may be linked to chronic health problems, but there is an over-representation from suicide, more commonly seen where there is a significant impact from comorbidities and mental health difficulties. There is also a link with social deprivation (again analogous to epilepsy) and to adverse childhood experiences.

Despite tic disorders being a common condition with significant effects on physical and mental health, there is no structure in the NHS for how these adult patients are managed. Many district general hospital adult neurology departments may have a consultant who specialises in movement disorders, but they may focus on conditions like Parkinson's or Huntington's and may not accept referrals for Tourette's. The patient with Tourette's and its attendant complications may have to travel a long way to see specialists in tertiary centres. This discrepancy and deficiency in the system is being highlighted by charities and patient advocacy groups.

Further reading

American Academy of Neurology (2019). Practice guideline recommendations: treatment of tics in people with Tourette syndrome and chronic tic disorders. https://www.aan.com/Guidelines/home/GuidelineDetail/958

Behring, E., Farhat, L.C., Landeros-Weisenburger, A., and Bloch, M.H. (2022). Meta-analysis: efficacy and tolerability of vesicular monoamine transporter type 2 inhibitors in the treatment of tic disorders. *Movement Disorders* 37 (4): 684–693.

Cavanna, A. (2020). *Pharmacological Treatment of Tics*. Cambridge: Cambridge University Press.

Dyke, K., Jackson, G., and Jackson, S. (2022). Non-invasive brain stimulation as therapy: systematic review and recommendations with a focus on the treatment of Tourette syndrome. *Experimental Brain Research* 240: 341–363.

Hollis, C., Pennant, M., Cuenca, J. et al. (2016). Clinical effectiveness and patient perspectives of different treatment strategies for tics in children and

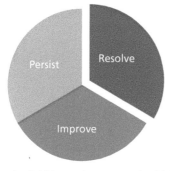

Figure 16.2 Prognosis of children and young people with Tourette's disorder.

adolescents with Tourette syndrome: a systematic review and qualitative analysis. *Health Technology Assessment* 20 (4): 1–496.

Jankovic, J., Hallett, M., Okun, M.S. et al. (2021). *Principles and Practice of Movement Disorders*, 3e. London: Elsevier.

Malmivaara, A. (2021). What is the effect of pharmacological treatment for attention deficit/hyperactivity disorder in children with comorbid tic disorders? A Cochrane review summary with commentary. *Developmental Medicine & Child Neurology* 63 (1): 14–15.

Müller-Vahl, K.R., Szejko, N., Verdellen, C. et al. (2022). European clinical guidelines for Tourette syndrome and other tic disorders: summary statement. *European Child and Adolescent Psychiatry* 31 (3): 377–382.

National Institute for Health and Care Excellence (NICE) (2019). Attention deficit hyperactivity disorder: diagnosis and management. NICE guideline [NG87]. https://www.nice.org.uk/guidance/ng87

National Institute for Health and Care Excellence (NICE) (2023). British National Formulary for Children (BNFC). https://bnfc.nice.org.uk/

Pringsheim, T., Okun, M.S., Muller-Vah, K. et al. (2019). Practice guideline recommendations summary: treatment of tics in people with Tourette syndrome and chronic tic disorders. *Neurology* 92: 896–906.

Pringsheim, T. and Piacentini, J. (2022). Internet based cognitive behavioural therapy for Tourette syndrome – meaningfully improving access to behavioural therapy for tics. *JAMA Network Open* 5 (8): 1–3.

Seideman, M.F. and Seideman, T.A. (2020). A review of the current treatment of Tourette syndrome. *Journal of Pediatric Pharmacology & Therapeutics* 25 (5): 401–412.

Taylor, E., Anderson, S., and Davies, E.B. (2022). 'I'm in pain and I want help': an online survey investigating the experiences of tic-related pain and use of pain management techniques in people with tics and tic disorders. *Frontiers in Psychiatry* 13: 1–15.

CHAPTER 17

An Introduction to Developmental Coordination Disorder

Munib Haroon

> **OVERVIEW**
>
> - Developmental coordination disorder (DCD) is characterised by a delay in the development of – or ongoing difficulties with – motor skills which interfere with activities of daily living and which arise during childhood, and for which there is no better alternative explanation.
> - DCD has a prevalence of <5–6% in children.
> - Genetic and environmental risk factors are well known, and DCD is associated with a number of other neurodevelopmental conditions.
> - DCD is associated with a number of physical and mental health conditions, the primary trigger for which may be the altered motor control itself.
> - The features of DCD are known to persist into adulthood.

Developmental coordination disorder (DCD) is characterised by four components (Figure 17.1). Firstly, a person's motor skills either develop slowly or continue to lag behind their chronological age (this does assume that it is not because of insufficient opportunity to learn such skills). This could involve delay with gross motor skills such as crawling (which could present with the use of alternate modes of locomotion, such as bottom shuffling), walking, running, riding a bike or delay with fine motor skills such as learning to write or to use utensils, scissors or doing up buttons, zips and laces. (DSM-5-TR does not specify types of DCD, but either gross or fine motor skill impairments may predominate). Secondly, the motor difficulties are significant and persistent and interfere with activities of daily living. In older children and adults this could manifest as difficulties with using a keyboard or learning to play a musical instrument or driving a car. Thirdly, the symptoms develop during childhood (although they may not be identified as having been present until adolescence or adulthood). Finally, the deficits observed cannot be better explained by an alternative medical explanation – such as intellectual developmental disorder, visual impairment or a neurological disorder that affects movement, such as cerebral palsy or muscular dystrophy – or a non-medical cause, such as social/cultural factors.

There is a lot of overlap between the term DCD and the term 'dyspraxia'; however, international consensus on how the latter term should be applied does not exist and so it is probably best avoided.

Epidemiology

The prevalence of DCD is hard to pinpoint. In the United Kingdom 1.8% of 7-year-olds had a diagnosis of DCD according to one study (with a further 3% having probable DCD, with related day-to-day issues suggestive of the disorder). Prevalence rates are higher in other countries, ranging from 7% to 9% in Canada, Sweden and Taiwan. Something close to 5–6% seems to be frequently quoted, but estimates range from 0.8% to 20%. This variation is possibly a function of case ascertainment and how the condition is defined in studies, but the condition is also known to be under-diagnosed on a day-to-day basis, and there is likely to be a geographical variation in clinician knowledge about the condition. The male : female ratio ranges from 2:1 to 7:1.

Aetiology

As with many neurodevelopmental conditions, there seems to be a genetic and environmental basis for DCD. The condition is associated with prematurity and low birthweight, but there also seem to be susceptibility genes for DCD, including genes shared with other co-occurring neurodevelopmental conditions (Box 17.1). Evidence from neuroimaging studies shows that children with DCD have differences in brain structure and function when compared to peers with more typical motor development patterns.

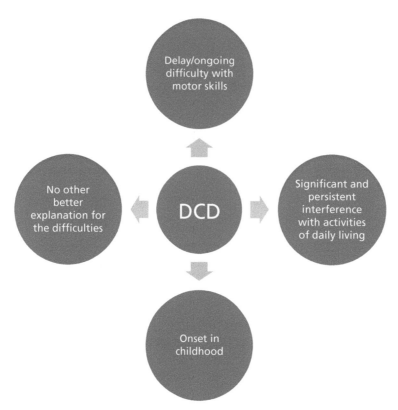

Figure 17.1 Developmental coordination disorder (DCD) is characterised by four essential components.

Box 17.1 **Claude**

Claude is 8 years old. He is seeing a paediatrician for suspected DCD. There is a strong family history of DCD; he has two brothers with the condition and his father notes that he had similar issues as a child. Claude cannot yet do shoelaces or ride a bike. He struggles with handwriting and has started to use a laptop at school. Claude was a late walker. The paediatrician notes that he was also premature and spent a month on the neonatal unit. As one of the first steps, the paediatrician contacts the neonatal unit to obtain Claude's discharge summary.

Box 17.2 **Jimmy**

Jimmy is 14. He was diagnosed with DCD when he was 9, but has had motor issues since he was a younger child. When he went to high school he experienced some bullying and a lot of teasing during sports, and although he was enthusiastic about football, he reports feeling as if he was hounded out of trying to play in the school team. This seemed to heighten his shyness and social difficulties (he was assessed for possible autism but did not meet the criteria) and he now reports feeling sad and isolated. The recent Covid-19 pandemic seemed to heighten these feelings.

Associated conditions

As well as an association with other neurodevelopmental conditions, DCD is associated with other physical health issues such as being overweight or obese, joint hypermobility, reduced physical fitness and decreased participation in physical and social activities. Children, young people and adults with DCD are also at risk for mental health difficulties, including difficulties with peers and depressive symptoms (Box 17.2). It is possible that the primary stressor for many of these physical and mental health issues is the motor coordination difficulty, whose presence leads to a cascade of effects. This has been termed the environmental stress hypothesis (Figure 17.2).

Adulthood and developmental coordination disorder

DCD in adults has not been as well studied as it has been in children, but studies show that the symptoms of DCD persist into adulthood (perhaps in 50–70% of cases), as do many of the associated conditions; for example, adults with DCD report significantly high levels of mental health difficulties. This can have implications for the same sorts of activities of daily living as it does in adolescence, but also on outcomes for independent living and employment, and may also affect the ability to perform important skills in adulthood like driving.

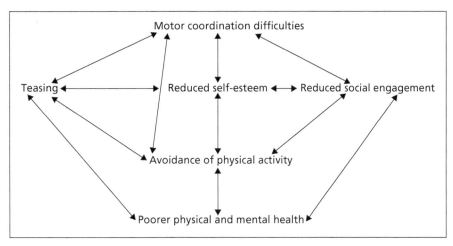

Figure 17.2 The primary stressor for the physical and mental health problems seen in developmental coordination disorder may be altered motor control, which sets up a range of effects.

Further reading

American Psychiatric Association (2022). *Diagnostic and Statistical Manual of Mental Disorders*, 5e. Text Revision. Washington, DC: American Psychiatric Association Publishing.

Blank, R., Barnett, A.L., Cairney, J. et al. (2019). International clinical practice recommendations on the definition, diagnosis, assessment, intervention, and psychosocial aspects of developmental coordination disorder. *Developmental Medicine and Child Neurology* 61: 242–285. https://doi.org/10.1111/dmcn.14132.

Gentle, J., Brady, D., Woodger, N. et al. (2021). Driving skills of individuals with and without developmental coordination disorder (DCD/dyspraxia). *Frontiers in Human Neuroscience* 15: 635649. https://doi.org/10.3389/fnhum.2021.635649.

Harris, S.R., Mickelson, E.C.R., and Zwicker, J.G. (2015). Diagnosis and management of developmental coordination disorder. *Canadian Medical Association Journal* 187 (9): 659–665.

CHAPTER 18

The Assessment and Diagnosis of Developmental Coordination Disorder

Munib Haroon

OVERVIEW

- The assessment for developmental coordination disorder (DCD) consists of obtaining a parental/patient history, gathering information from other sources, carrying out a physical examination and conducting an objective test of motor performance.

- A diagnosis in under 5s may be unreliable.

- There is no role for screening to enable early diagnosis.

- There may be a need for formal cognitive tests as part of the assessment.

- Assessment should try to determine whether DCD is the best diagnosis, or whether the presentation may be due to something else and whether there may be other coexisting conditions.

- DCD can be assessed and diagnosed in adults.

Assessment of developmental coordination disorder

A child or young person may be referred for an assessment because of problems arising at home, school or work. There is a wide variation in when children acquire motor skills, so when issues are noted there may be a period of monitoring before a child is referred on for further assessment. There may be some variation in local assessment pathways, but generally in the United Kingdom an assessment for DCD will require input from a therapist (occupational therapy or physiotherapy) and a doctor.

As with many conditions, early identification can allow earlier intervention. This raises the question of screening. Screening, however, requires the presence of reliable, valid, acceptable, cost-effective and time-efficient tools. Owing to a lack of such instruments, screening remains problematic. Similarly, while making a diagnosis as early as possible in life seems sensible, there are problems with such an approach. As a result, trying to make a diagnosis in children under 5 is often not advised (Box 18.1).

The diagnostic assessment is concerned with assessing the duration, extent, pattern and severity of motor function issues and in doing so ensuring that DCD is the most appropriate diagnosis; that is, making sure that the pattern of features and how they have developed is consistent with DCD and that an alternative diagnosis is not likely (Figure 18.1).

The diagnosis of DCD is a clinical one. It involves the traditional medical approaches of obtaining a history (Box 18.2) and examining the child (Box 18.3), but in addition it is important to assess information from sources other than the parent/child, especially the school. Information can be in the form of freehand reports, questionnaires or a combination, and should detail motor function, cognitive function/academic achievements, behavioural issues and concerns about DCD and other neurodevelopmental conditions. In the author's experience, this information is generally most efficiently collected prior to seeing the child. Assessing cognition is important, but where a school does not have concerns about this, formalised testing will probably not be required.

Assessment also involves the use of standardised tests of motor function, and these are typically the domain of an occupational therapist/physiotherapist. Examples of well-validated tools include Movement Assessment Battery for Children—Second Edition (MABC-2) and Bruininks-Oseretsky Test of Motor Proficiency Second Edition (BOT-2). These tests have sensitivities below 90% and may 'miss' approximately 10% of children presenting with features of DCD. As such, where a child has features of DCD and does not meet the criteria for diagnosis on one test (e.g. motor function <16th centile), current recommendations are that a second test should be considered, or a second assessment be carried out by another expert.

Any concerns around visual/neurological features not associated with DCD on history/examination should prompt investigation into other disorders, and the presence of a learning disability should raise the question of whether the motor difficulties are in keeping with the child's intellectual development (which would not lead to diagnosing DCD) or whether they are even more delayed than intellectual development (which in theory could still lead to a diagnosis of DCD).

Clinical features

The features of DCD vary widely and with age. There may be a delay in achieving motor milestones, although many children with DCD achieve these at a normal age. Non-motor milestones should be normal – if not, this should suggest that either an alternative diagnosis should be explored or that a comorbidity might be present. A variety of skills may be delayed, both fine motor (such as writing) and gross motor (such as throwing a ball). Difficulties may be seen/experienced as an impairment in carrying out a task or as marked slowness. For example, when handwriting is affected this may involve both legibility and the speed at which the affected individual writes.

Some children with DCD show additional motor activity such as choreiform movements of unsupported limbs and also mirror movements. The role of these in making a diagnosis is unclear.

It is important to be alert to features suggestive of other physical and neurodevelopmental conditions or of psychological problems. Children and young people with DCD may be at greater risk of having low self-esteem or being victimised by others. While DCD is primarily a motor problem, the presence of other biological and environmental factors may have consequences for wider aspects of a child/young person's mental/physical health.

Other investigations

Standardised testing to assess the degree of motor difficulty is part of the core assessment and sometimes there may be a need to formally assess a child's intellectual functioning. There is, however,

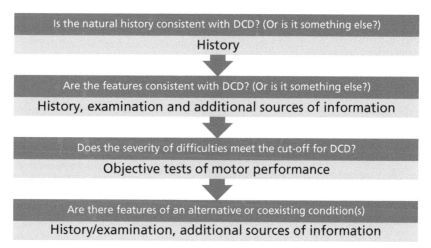

Figure 18.1 Assessment of developmental coordination disorder (DCD).

Box 18.2 **Areas to enquire about when taking a medical history for DCD**

- History of presenting complaint. This would include obtaining information about the duration of the problems, their extent and enquiring about ADL: self-care (such as using buttons/zips/washing/dressing), activities at school during formal lessons (such as using a keyboard, writing, doing sport) and outside, such as leisure/vocational pastimes (e.g. swimming, riding a bike, catching/kicking balls). It is important to take cultural factors into account.
- Previous medical history. This should start with maternal pregnancy, including the use of substances, delivery and associated complications, early illness and conditions, as well as information about injuries (accidental and non-accidental) and possible/confirmed neurological disorders and psychiatric disorders.
- Review of systems. A general review should be considered to enable a clinician to think about broader neurological presentations and also possible psychiatric/psychological presentations and other neurodevelopmental conditions that commonly co-occur.
- Developmental history. This should cover a child/person's entire lifespan and address both motor and non-motor issues such as language and socialisation/communication. Obtaining an accurate history of earlier development can become more difficult with age.
- Educational history. This should enquire about progress from nursery onwards, noting progress, achievement, concerns and supportive measures, such as Education, Health and Care plans (EHCPs), one-to-one teaching and the use of other supportive measures such as extra time during exams/tests or the use of keyboards. Input from therapists at school should be requested too.
- Family/social history. As well as information on neurological, psychiatric and neurodevelopmental conditions in the family, it is important to ask about the structure of the family, socioeconomic status and involvement with social care.

no role for routine investigations to rule out other medical conditions. Blood tests such as creatine kinase would be carried out if there was a concern around muscular dystrophy, and magnetic resonance imaging (MRI) of the brain might be required if there were concerns around cerebral palsy. Referrals for visual assessment might be required in individual cases, depending on the specific concerns.

Finalising a diagnosis

Pathways will vary, but a number of different professionals may be involved, such as a physiotherapist/occupational therapist and a paediatrician. Concluding a diagnosis can often involve a shared discussion or a professional assessing the child with the results of other assessments in hand, and determining if the child or young person fulfils the DSM-5-TR (or ICD-11) criteria for DCD.

Developmental coordination disorder in adults

DSM-5-TR mentions adults in relation to the same set of criteria for DCD, and the European Academy of Childhood Disability (see Further Reading) has adapted these for use in adults, by modifying some of the DSM's terminology in relation to ADL. For example, in adults, as well as asking about ADL that overlap with those of childhood, it will be important to enquire about a different/broader range of difficulties. These may be vocational and be related to specific aspects of a job, related to doing DIY and chores, or to other essential skills such as driving.

While diagnostic schemes are not a barrier to diagnosis in adults, the lack of adult services may be an impediment and may vary greatly from country to country, and even from region to region in the United Kingdom. The pathways leading to a diagnosis in adulthood may also be broader, for example where difficulties are identified at work or at university, an initial assessment may be carried out by an occupational therapist, psychologist or educational psychologist. Although the principles of assessment in adulthood are similar to those in childhood – history, gathering information, conducting an examination and performing other criteria-referenced assessments, such as those of motor performance – there are a limited number of standardised, validated assessments for adults at this point in time.

Further reading

American Psychiatric Association (2022). *Diagnostic and Statistical Manual of Mental Disorders*, 5e. Text Revision. Washington, DC: American Psychiatric Association Publishing.

Blank, R., Barnett, A.L., Cairney, J. et al. (2019). International clinical practice recommendations on the definition, diagnosis, assessment, intervention, and psychosocial aspects of developmental coordination disorder. *Developmental Medicine and Child Neurology* 61: 242–285. https://doi.org/10.1111/dmcn.14132.

Harris, S.R., Mickelson, E.C.R., and Zwicker, J.G. (2015). Diagnosis and management of developmental coordination disorder. *Canadian Medical Association Journal* 187 (9): 659–665.

CHAPTER 19

Treatment and Interventions for Developmental Coordination Disorder

Munib Haroon

> **OVERVIEW**
>
> - A diagnosis of developmental coordination disorder (DCD) in children and young people will often necessitate some degree of intervention.
> - As well as interventions for the motor aspects of DCD, children and young people with DCD may require intervention for physical and mental health and associated neurodevelopmental conditions. They may also require support for social concerns, whether at home or school.
> - There are two broad interventional approaches for DCD: body function-oriented and activity-oriented.
> - Improving fitness may represent a 'triple win', with better motor control and also improved mental and physical well-being.

When a child's motor function necessitates a diagnosis of developmental coordination disorder (DCD), it is likely that interventions of some kind will be required.

Interventions for DCD should consider a child's difficulties and strengths, while noting the environments or contexts in which difficulties occur. Ideally a holistic assessment will allow a broad approach to support. A child with DCD may have other physical, mental or neurodevelopmental conditions requiring guidance and support (Figure 19.1). They may also have other social needs, and so may require intervention from a broad range of professionals, including therapy services (physiotherapy/occupational therapy), paediatrics, Child and Adolescent Mental Health Services (CAMHS), social services, educational psychology and teachers.

In all of this, it is important to take into account the needs, desires and goals of the child/young person and their families.

Interventions for developmental coordination disorder

For some children with DCD, adjustments to the surrounding environment may be all that are required to support the motor difficulties/delays.

Support may be required for fine motor aspects such as writing, using cutlery or doing buttons and laces, or for more gross motor-related tasks such as walking, running or activities requiring greater levels of coordination and balance.

Activity-oriented and body function-oriented approaches

There are two traditional approaches to interventions for DCD. Those that focus on targeting the underlying basis of performance issues are denoted body function-oriented approaches, while those that target specific areas of difficulty are termed activity-oriented approaches (Figure 19.2).

The British Association of Childhood Disability's (BACD) recent European guidance on DCD recommends activity/participation-oriented approaches primarily; this is on the basis of evidence from meta-analyses of randomised controlled trial (RCT) data. Such approaches focus on activities of daily living, including personal care, play, leisure/sports, arts and crafts, academic and vocational tasks. It is recommended that such interventions try to generalise across different activities and environmental contexts, and that they aim to involve family, teachers or other significant parties who can promote opportunities for practice/performance across a wide area of activities. This is not to say that there is supportive evidence from meta-analyses, or even single RCTs, for every type of such intervention (for example, the evidence for handwriting training and teaching keyboarding skills early on for children with handwriting difficulties is not as robust; Box 19.1), but accumulating evidence points towards such approaches tending to work better than others.

Activity-oriented approaches may involve breaking down complicated activities or tasks – which a child finds difficult – into a series of smaller steps, which can be practised individually and on a regular basis. Adaptations and aids, such as pen grips or specially adapted computer mouses, may help with activities like writing and computing.

The promotion of body function-oriented approaches in the past has been based on the idea that improving body function (with respect to motor control or proprioception) will make specific tasks

---

ABC of Neurodevelopmental Disorders, First Edition. Edited by Munib Haroon.
© 2024 John Wiley & Sons Ltd. Published 2024 by John Wiley & Sons Ltd.

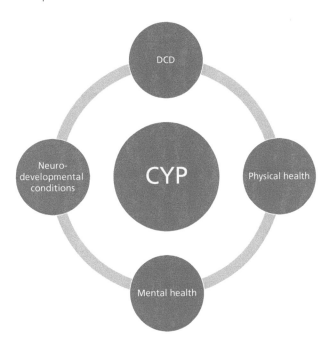

Figure 19.1 The child or young person (CYP) with developmental coordination disorder (DCD) may require a number of different health-related interventions. This will include addressing the core features of DCD, but may also necessitate addressing other aspects of mental or physical well-being as well as the presence of other neurodevelopmental conditions.

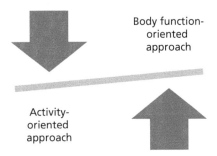

Figure 19.2 There are two broad approaches to interventions for development coordination disorder (DCD): those that focus on the underlying basis of performance issues (body function-oriented approach) and those that focus on specific areas of difficulty (activity-oriented approach).

Box 19.1 **Tommy**

Tommy, 8 years old, has ongoing difficulties with his handwriting despite having had handwriting training. He has been taught keyboarding skills and has a laptop to use at school and for homework. While this helps, he still finds it difficult to produce written work and it is likely that he will need extra time during exams.

easier. While there is some evidence supporting this, it remains limited, and the BACD recommends that such approaches, when used, stay close to or directly address the actual activities that there is a wish to be improved.

There is also evidence suggesting a role for other 'adjuncts' such as video games training and interventions to improve

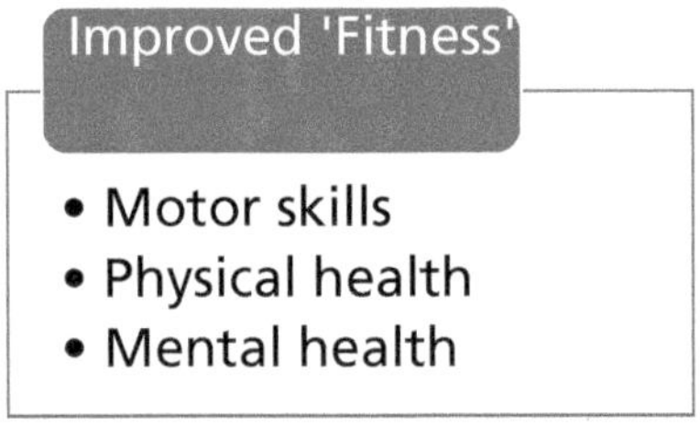

Improved 'Fitness'

- Motor skills
- Physical health
- Mental health

Figure 19.3 Exercise/physical activity may provide a 'triple win' by helping to improve motor skills, but also helping to improve physical and mental well-being.

general fitness. Improved general fitness (Figure 19.3) may also provide a triple win, not only helping to improve motor skills but also helping with aspects of physical health (e.g. excess weight gain) and mental health (e.g. symptoms of anxiety and low mood).

The setting in which interventions are performed is an important aspect to consider, as small group-based interventions may support the development of group dynamics and socialisation as well as targeting the core aspects of DCD; however, this may deter children who are especially anxious about their motor skills. More precise aspects to do with the forms of interventions, such as duration, frequency and content, remain unclear.

Adult interventions

Many of the principles already underlined in this chapter would seem to apply for adults. The core features of DCD may need support and should be addressed with an eye on the individual's difficulties, strengths, environment, goals, aspirations and priorities (see Box 19.2 and Figure 19.4). In addition, associated physical and mental health issues may require support, as may the presence of other neurodevelopmental conditions. There is limited evidence on the efficacy of particular individual approaches in adults, but the evidence base for activity-oriented approaches in children and young people would suggest that

Box 19.2 **Sarah**

Sarah, 24, is a foundation-year trainee in medicine. She was diagnosed with DCD and autism as a child, but managed with basic adaptations and by restricting what she did in her spare time. However, now she is seeking advice from a therapist because she has a number of goals and aspirations that she fears will be/are being impeded by her DCD. Her therapist identifies that passing her driving test is her greatest priority and together they identify that finding an instructor who has worked with similar individuals may be helpful, as may learning to drive an automatic car, and driving in low-stress conditions while she gets her confidence back. Her therapist discusses how a tennis serve can be modified and broken down into individual steps to be practised when alone and suggests finding a sympathetic cello teacher, reminding her that most adult learning of musical instrument happens one to one, not in a group. A discussion with occupational health, the college tutor and the Royal College of Surgeons is suggested as a first step, to identify reasonable adjustments and for career advice.

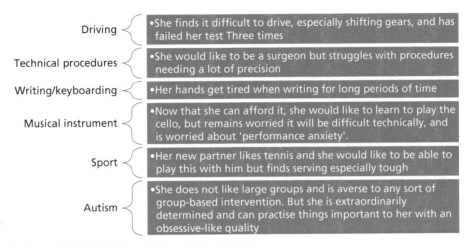

Figure 19.4 Support for Sarah, an adult with developmental coordination disorder.

such approaches may be more effective in adults when compared to body function-oriented approaches.

DCD can remain a significant issue for those affected by it as adults. It may impede many activities of daily living and life, and its significance should not be trivialised.

Further reading

American Psychiatric Association (2022). *Diagnostic and Statistical Manual of Mental Disorders*, 5e. Text Revision. Washington, DC: American Psychiatric Association Publishing.

Blank, R., Barnett, A.L., Cairney, J. et al. (2019). International clinical practice recommendations on the definition, diagnosis, assessment, intervention, and psychosocial aspects of developmental coordination disorder. *Developmental Medicine and Child Neurology* 61: 242–285. https://doi.org/10.1111/dmcn.14132.

Gentle, J., Brady, D., Woodger, N. et al. (2021). Driving skills of individuals with and without developmental coordination disorder (DCD/dyspraxia). *Frontiers in Human Neuroscience* 15: 635649. https://doi.org/10.3389/fnhum.2021.635649.

Harris, S.R., Mickelson, E.C.R., and Zwicker, J.G. (2015). Diagnosis and management of developmental coordination disorder. *Canadian Medical Association Journal* 187 (9): 659–665.

CHAPTER 20

An Introduction to Specific Learning Disorder

Tracy Laverick and Julie Armstrong

OVERVIEW

- Specific learning disorder is a common neurodevelopmental disorder with a prevalence of around 10% of the population.
- It is defined as a difficulty in the acquisition of academic skills, namely reading, writing and arithmetic.
- There is no cure, but appropriate intervention and support can ameliorate the impact and enable individuals to have successful careers.

Definition

Specific learning disorder (SpLD) is a common neurodevelopmental condition that presents as difficulties in learning specific academic skills, namely reading, spelling, writing processes and arithmetic (Table 20.1). The difficulties must be persistent, despite intervention targeting the particular area(s) of difficulty. Given that the acquisition of different academic skills can be affected, it can be considered to be a group of disorders, rather than a single one, with different terms given to each specific area of difficulty.

The terms commonly used within the United Kingdom are:

- Dyslexia – inaccurate reading and/or spelling difficulties at word level.
- Dysgraphia – difficulty in spelling and organisation of writing, including grammar and punctuation.
- Dyscalculia – inaccurate calculation, number awareness and difficulty in retaining arithmetic facts.

While these may appear to be three very separate difficulties, the overlapping of different features of each, particularly when considering secondary difficulties (see Chapter 21), makes the general term specific learning disorder more appropriate; however, there is a tension around the definition in that it does not recognise which specific element of academic skill the person is having difficulty in acquiring.

History

First identified in Germany in 1877, dyslexia had its roots in ophthalmology, when it was observed that some adult patients had difficulty in reading printed text. The term 'word blindness' was coined for this, and later 'dyslexia' came into use to bring it into line with other contemporary medical conditions that described similar difficulties. In the first half of the twentieth century, research into cerebral dominance moved dyslexia into the world of cognitive development.

By the 1960s and 1970s, dyslexia was firmly established. However, there was much controversy, some of which still persists, around it being a 'middle-class' disease, used by middle-class parents to explain poor academic performance in their offspring. There was also a tendency at the time for a discrepancy model of diagnosis to be used, with children who were otherwise intelligent but who struggled with reading and spelling labelled 'dyslexic'. Ironically, performance in mathematics was often used as the comparison, although it is now accepted that while 10% of people with dyslexia are good at mathematics, 40% will also struggle with it.

Dyscalculia was first recognised as early as 1919, with the term being used from the 1940s onwards, though it is widely accepted that it was first described as a learning disability as late as 1974. Dysgraphia was first studied as an entity in its own right in the 1960s, when areas of difficulty within writing were discovered that were not readily explained as dyslexia.

Into the twenty-first century, SpLDs are widely recognised and accepted within education as a special educational need, requiring support that is 'additional to and different from' (Department of Education/Department of Health 2015) that required by neurotypical peers.

Epidemiology

SpLD is thought to affect around 10% of the population, and around 4% are thought to be severely affected. The prevalence of boys to girls is in a ratio of 3:1.

ABC of Neurodevelopmental Disorders, First Edition. Edited by Munib Haroon.
© 2024 John Wiley & Sons Ltd. Published 2024 by John Wiley & Sons Ltd.

Table 20.1 Specific learning disorders overview.

Dyslexia	Dysgraphia	Dyscalculia
Inaccurate reading and/or spelling difficulties at word level	Difficulty in spelling and organisation of writing, including grammar and punctuation	Inaccurate calculation, number awareness and difficulty in retaining arithmetic facts

Aetiology

The exact cause is unknown. Premature birth and very low birthweight increase the risk of SpLD. There is also thought to be a genetic element, certainly in regard to dyslexia, as reading difficulties tend to run in families. While the genetic factor is widely accepted, there is probably an additional environmental factor at play in that a parent with dyslexia is less likely to be able to support a child with reading and spelling tasks at home.

While SpLD cannot be cured, there are certain protective factors that can be put in place that are supportive. Having good language skills is seen as a protective feature, as is early identification of difficulties.

Key features

All SpLDs are underpinned by four common features:
- Weak working memory
- Persistent difficulty in spite of appropriate intervention
- Slowness to automaticity
- Can occur across the intellectual range
  These occur in the absence of:
- Visual or hearing impairment
- Mental disorders
- Neurological disorders
- Psychosocial difficulty
- Language differences
- Lack of adequate opportunities to acquire the skills

Prognosis and outcomes

While SpLD is incurable, good-quality intervention, including the use of assistive technology, can enable individuals to achieve good academic outcomes. Having this condition is not a barrier to a successful life for many (Box 20.1).

In 2014, a book entitled *The Dyslexia Debate* pointed out the while individuals might experience difficulties due to the constraints of the education system, there are other traits that can provide an advantage in certain professions and areas of life. For example, while 10% of the general population has SpLD, that figure rises to 29% of Royal College of Art students with an SpLD.

Further reading

Butterworth, B. (2019). *Dyscalculia, from Science to Education*. London: Routledge.

Department for Education/Department for Health (2015). Special educational needs and disability code of practice: 0-25 years. Statutory guidance for organisations which work with and support children and young people who have special educational needs or disabilities. https://assets.publishing.service.gov.uk/government/uploads/system/uploads/attachment_data/file/398815/SEND_Code_of_Practice_January_2015.pdf

Elliott, J. and Grigorenko, E. (2014). *The Dyslexia Debate*. Cambridge: Cambridge University Press.

Rapp, B. and McCloskey, M. (ed.) (2018). *Developmental Dysgraphia*. London: Routledge.

Reid, G. (2016). *Dyslexia: A Practitioner's Handbook*, 5e. Hoboken, NJ: Wiley-Blackwell.

Snowling, M.J. (2019). *Dyslexia: A Very Short Introduction*. Oxford: Oxford University Press.

CHAPTER 21

The Assessment and Diagnosis of Specific Learning Disorder in Children and Young People

Tracy Laverick and Julie Armstrong

> **OVERVIEW**
>
> - Any assessment of specific learning disorder (SpLD) needs to be informed by parental concerns, access to educational opportunities, intervention to address areas of difficulty and progress from these interventions.
> - Assessments are completed by a professional with additional qualifications in SpLD or by an educational/child psychologist.
> - Severe difficulties may require education staff to request additional resources to meet their needs.

Children are brought in to see their family doctor when a parent, guardian or teacher is concerned that the child may be having difficulties acquiring reading, writing or mathematical skills and that this might be the sign of a specific learning disability. This can be the case if the parent themselves has a specific learning disorder (SpLD) or there is a wider family history of SpLD. The parent may reflect on how this experience was for them and be concerned that their child will have a similar, potentially negative, experience. The NHS in England does not provide assessments for SpLDs, but it is valuable to be aware of the DSM-5 assessment criteria, the process of assessment and support available for families.

Family members may have concerns around the child's learning prior to age 7, and there is still considerable variation in children's abilities to acquire reading, writing and mathematical skills at this age. Identification of needs, additional support and interventions should be put in place in the early years, but formal diagnosis is not recommended prior to 7 years of age. Difficulties become increasingly apparent within the later primary years as the child struggles to develop specific learning skills and the gap between them and their peers widens.

When a child is brought to see a health professional because of concerns around SpLD, it is important to be aware of the child's strengths as well as areas of difficulty. It is important to identify if the family have spoken to the educational setting around their concerns and which interventions and provision have been put into place. If the child is home educated, the parent should be able to share which evidence-based systematic interventions have been put in place and their child's progress in these.

The Special Educational Needs and Disabilities Code of Practice (2015) stipulates a graduated response to a child's needs by education staff. There should be a process of Assess–Plan–Do–Review (Figure 21.1) in place, with levels of support increasing if the child is not making progress. Every educational setting must have a qualified teacher as a special educational needs coordinator (SENCO), whose role it is to identify children's learning needs and oversee the interventions and support required for them to make progress. School staff should create a support plan for the child's needs, the support they require and their progress. This must be created alongside parents, so they are fully informed of what is in place for their child within the setting. It may be that families bring such documentation to their consultation appointment.

SpLDs are to be viewed as on a continuum. Those that have a mild to moderate impact on daily functioning and access to education would be expected to be supported by staff in school, with or without a formal diagnosis. Only those children whose difficulties are having a severe impact on their daily functioning would be able to access external professional support and potentially a formal diagnosis.

Additional assessment and support may be offered, in some areas, through advisory teacher services, accessed via the school and coordinated by the SENCO. These advisory services can provide assessments and recommendations for meeting children's learning needs. In areas where such support is not available, school SENCOs may be able to refer to their local Educational Psychology Service if the child's needs are severe.

Parents can source screening and diagnosis of SpLD using private assessment services. This assessment may include a family history and the child's responses within assessment and should be administered by either an Health and Care Professions Council (HCPC) Registered Educational Psychologist or a professional with an Assessment Practising Certificate issued by the Specialist Assessments Standards Committee (SASC). If the private assessment identifies mild to moderate needs, it would continue to be expected that these needs would be met from within the school's resources and the Assess–Plan–Do–Review process.

ABC of Neurodevelopmental Disorders, First Edition. Edited by Munib Haroon.
© 2024 John Wiley & Sons Ltd. Published 2024 by John Wiley & Sons Ltd.

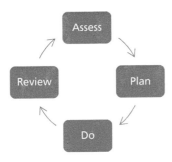

Figure 21.1 The Assess–Plan–Do–Review cycle.

When having the initial GP consultation, it is important to get the family history of learning needs, including the family's exposure to books and reading materials. Parents may be anxious regarding diagnosis due to their own SpLD needs and children may have experienced limited access to reading materials/numeracy support due to this anxiety.

Assessment criteria

Although there are multiple assessment criteria for SpLD, there are aspects that are common. First, assessment must show that the child has difficulties with learning and academic skills in at least one of the following areas: inaccurate or slow/effortful reading; comprehension; spelling; written expression; mastering number sense, number facts or calculation; or mathematical reasoning (see Figure 21.2). There may be individual criteria for each of these areas, for example dyslexia or dyscalculia.

Secondly, these difficulties should be substantially below the expected achievement level for the individual's chronological age and have a significant impact on their academic performance or with daily living skills.

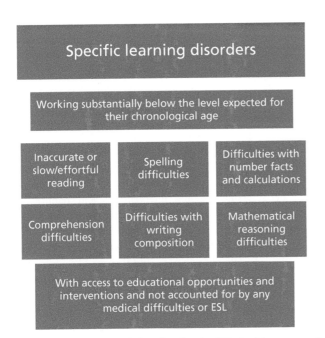

Figure 21.2 Features of specific learning disorders (ESL, English as a second language).

Box 21.1 **The rose report definition of dyslexia**

- Dyslexia is a learning difficulty that primarily affects the skills involved in accurate and fluent word reading and spelling
- Characteristic features of dyslexia are difficulties in phonological awareness, verbal memory and verbal processing speed
- Dyslexia occurs across the range of intellectual abilities
- It is best thought of as a continuum, not a distinct category, and there are no clear cut-off points
- Co-occurring difficulties may be seen in aspects of language, motor coordination, mental calculation, concentration and personal organisation, but these are not, by themselves, markers of dyslexia
- A good indication of the severity and persistence of dyslexic difficulties can be gained by examining how the individual responds or has responded to well-founded interventions

Source: Adapted from Rose (2009).

Thirdly, these difficulties must be observed during school age (7–18 years old), but may not be identified until they leave formal schooling and the academic demands exceed their skills. Assessment is not recommended prior to the age of 7, as there is a wide variation in skills up to this point that may not be indicative of a long-term pervasive disorder, and within some cultures children do not access formal reading instruction until that age.

Finally, the assessment must consider whether the difficulties experienced are best described as linked to other intellectual, sensory, medical or neurological disorders in the first instance. A full history is required to ensure that difficulties are not due to adversity, English as a second language (ESL), a lack of educational instruction or access to intervention. If an alternative explanation for the child's needs is evident, then an SpLD diagnosis may not be appropriate.

The assessment process should identify if these aspects are met and identify each of the individual areas of difficulty experienced. A synthesis of information from the individual's history, information from education staff and an educational assessment are required for diagnosis. The assessment criteria detailed are applicable to both literacy- and numeracy-based disorders.

The British Dyslexia Association and education-based professionals often use the Rose report definition (2009) of dyslexia as their assessment criteria (see Box 21.1)

Specialist assessment

A specific learning difficulties assessment can be carried out by a range of staff with specialist training in SpLD or by an educational psychologist (Box 21.2). Local authority areas and professionals may differ in the terminology used, tending to prefer the use of

Box 21.2 **Who can assess for specific learning disorders?**

Assessment can be completed by:
- Education professionals with additional, formal training in SpLD
- Educational and/or child psychologists

specific learning difficulties as opposed to dyslexia, dyscalculia, dysgraphia or SpLD. Labels such as SpLD can be less understood by school staff and parents due to the familiarity with and broader understanding of the terms dyslexia and dyscalculia.

Assessment for an SpLD occurs after children have had regular access to learning opportunities and interventions, so poor or irregular access to educational opportunities would need to be addressed before interventions can be implemented and monitored and a diagnosis given. Assessment and diagnosis are usually completed by education-based teams due to the requirement of educational progress being monitored following appropriate intervention or by a private organisation or individual.

Frustrations can occur for families due to the amount of time the process can take, and the requirement to gain assessment and intervention through educational settings, and this may, in turn, lead to families seeking a medical solution. It is important to discuss with the family the communication between them and education staff and review how needs are currently being addressed.

Assessment tools

There is considerable variation in how SpLD is identified within each local authority area, and the assessment used may vary by practitioner and the training they have received. Some of the assessment tools used by professionals include:
- Clinical Evaluation of Language Fundamentals–5 (CELF-5)
- Phonological Assessment Battery (PhAB 2)
- Comprehensive Test of Phonological Processing–2 (CTOPP-2)
- York Assessment of Reading Comprehension (YARC)
- Grey Oral Reading Test–5 (GORT-5)

Educational psychologists may use cognitive assessment batteries and restricted assessments such as:
- British Ability Scale 3 (BAS 3)
- Wechsler Intelligence Scale for Children (WISC V)
- Wechsler Individual Achievement Test (WIAT III)

Some non-specialist educators may use dyslexia screening tests. These may indicate the possibility of an SpLD but should not be treated as diagnostic, although they may indicate the need for further assessment or intervention.

Comorbidity and secondary factors

Children and young people with a diagnosis of SpLD may also be affected by a range of other factors that influence their ability to be able to manage within the educational environment. These include:
- Altered gross and/or fine motor skills
- Differences in organisational skills
- Reduced sequential memory
- Reduced working memory
- Confusing left from right
- Forgetting instructions
- Visual and auditory processing difficulties
- Fatigue from additional effort needed to keep up with reading/writing

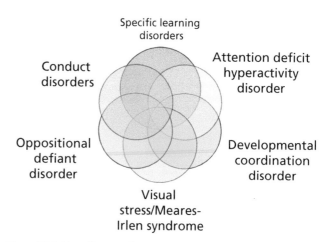

Figure 21.3 Venn diagram of comorbid factors.

Other comorbid conditions include (Figure 21.3):
- Attention deficit hyperactivity disorder (ADHD)
- Developmental coordination disorder (DCD)
- Visual stress/Meares-Irlen syndrome
- Oppositional defiant disorder (ODD)
- Conduct disorders

Children and young people with SpLD may be affected by mental health needs associated with difficulties in school, and be vulnerable to bullying. Additional factors might include:
- Lower self-esteem and not seeing themselves as a learner
- Anxiety when completing academic tasks
- Avoiding literacy/numeracy-based activities, which affects academic progress
- Poor motivation or inattention
- Becoming withdrawn or disruptive
- Becoming socially isolated

The psychological impact of SpLD should not be underestimated, as these children and young people are required to put in significant amounts of effort in everyday learning activities but continue to have increased difficulties; they may have taken part in continuous interventions but despite this experienced very limited educational success, within their area of difficulty.

It is predicted that up to 10% of the population may have SpLD, but that severity would follow the normal distribution. Up to 6% of SpLDs may be classified as mild when most needs are met by appropriate differentiation in the educational setting. If needs are identified as moderate, it would be expected that the individual would be accessing ongoing interventions and require some additional support within learning activities. At this level school staff can provide this from their delegated resources.

Up to 4% of children and young people with a diagnosis of SpLD will have needs classified as severe, and they are likely to require a high level of support with access to specialised teaching and interventions. They are also likely to require specialist equipment such as reading pens and access arrangements for exams and assessments. To provide this individualised level of support, the parent or school SENCO may wish to request an assessment for an Education Health and Care plan (EHCP).

If a young person goes to university and the demands of the curriculum exceed their capacity, they may be able to request an SpLD assessment through their university. Many universities offer additional student support for young people with SpLD and/or access to the Student Disability Allowance for additional equipment and support.

Further reading

British Dyslexia Association (2022). *The Dyslexia Handbook 2022*. Bracknell: BDA. www.bdadyslexia.org.uk/shop/books/the-dyslexia-handbook-2022

Department for Education and Department of Health (2015). Special educational needs and disability code of practice: 0 to 25 years. https://assets. publishing.service.gov.uk/media/5a7dcb85ed915d2ac884d995/ SEND_Code_of_Practice_January_2015.pdf

Rose, J. (2009). *Identifying and Teaching Children and Young People with Dyslexia and Literacy Difficulties*. Nottingham: DCSF.

SpLD Assessment Standards Committee (SASC) (2019). SASC guidance on assessment of dyslexia and maths difficulties within other specific learning difficulties. http://www.sasc.org.uk/media/3gtdmm0s/ assessment-of-dyscalculia-maths-sasc-nov-2019.pdf

CHAPTER 22

Specific Learning Disorder: Interventions and Management

Tracy Laverick and Julie Armstrong

> **OVERVIEW**
>
> - Interventions for specific learning disorders must be matched to the individual's profile of need.
> - Interventions should be evidence based, multisensory, structured, sequential and provide opportunities for over-learning.
> - Assistive technology should be considered to support access to wider learning.

Intervention as part of the diagnostic process

Part of the definition of specific learning disorder (SpLD) is that it is *persistent* despite the individual having had access to appropriate learning opportunities. Careful monitoring of the response to intervention is indicative of the severity of the disorder.

It is not uncommon for children to struggle with acquiring a particular aspect of learning from time to time, including those skills that might be indicative of an SpLD such as difficulties with reading, spelling or arithmetic. It is understandable that parents and educators will be concerned; however, there are so many factors that could contribute to these difficulties that it is not helpful to immediately assign a diagnosis of SpLD. Given the epidemiology of SpLD, most difficulties will be transitory in nature and will respond to good-quality intervention. It is only those with persistent difficulties that evidence would suggest require a formal diagnosis.

The purpose of intervention

It is important to remember that SpLDs are life-long conditions and cannot be cured. The purpose of intervention is to ameliorate the difficulties in acquiring specific skills.

Within a classroom setting, there are general measures that can be taken that will benefit learners with SpLDs. Changing the background colour of electronic whiteboards to a pastel colour has been found to stabilise text rather than it jumping around. Not requiring learners with SpLDs to read aloud to the class can reduce their anxiety and embarrassment. The use of planning grids and graphic organisers can support those with dysgraphia to structure their writing, while the use of concrete equipment to model arithmetical procedures can support understanding. All of these steps can be taken without requiring additional staffing or funding, and without any diagnosis.

Key principles of intervention

The MOSS acronym is a good starting point for the development of interventions (Table 22.1).

A 'little and often' approach to intervention delivery has also been found to be beneficial. Three 20-minute sessions across a week are more beneficial to the retention of skills than a single hour-long session in the week.

Use of teaching assistants

There is a common misconception that all children with special educational needs require an additional adult to sit with them to support them with their work. Research has shown that this is not the case and that it can be detrimental to the learner, in that the teaching assistant will often do the work for the young person and therefore learning does not take place. This creates a learned dependency. Working exclusively with a teaching assistant has also been shown to be a barrier to the young person collaborating with their peers.

Teaching assistants can be useful when they deliver evidence-based interventions, under the supervision of a teacher, for short periods of time. Teachers are best placed to identify gaps in learning and to match the intervention to the needs profile of the learner. They can also monitor progress and, if necessary, change the intervention if the child or young person is not making progress.

Which intervention?

Many interventions are available to purchase from educational publishers, particularly for dyslexia, though far fewer for dysgraphia and dyscalculia. It is important to ensure that the particular intervention chosen is matched to the specific difficulties being demonstrated by the individual learner.

ABC of Neurodevelopmental Disorders, First Edition. Edited by Munib Haroon.
© 2024 John Wiley & Sons Ltd. Published 2024 by John Wiley & Sons Ltd.

Table 22.1 The MOSS (Multisensory, Over-learning, Structured, Sequential) acronym for the development of interventions.

Multisensory	**O**ver-learning
Involves visual, auditory and kinaesthetic elements	Provides opportunities not just to learn a skill once, but to learn it repeatedly and to apply it
Structured	**S**equential
In which each session follows a given pattern, with change to the content only	Enables previous learning to be practised to ensure that it is firmly embedded, with the next piece of learning introduced alongside it

Tables 22.2–22.4 identify the key features of interventions for dyslexia, dysgraphia and dyscalculia, respectively. Where examples have been given, they are those that are commonly used in mainstream schools in the United Kingdom. As interventions need to be tailored to the learner's specific needs, it should be noted that these are not recommendations but indicative of interventions that may support learners. The learner's response to an intervention must be carefully monitored and the work adapted or an alternative intervention employed as necessary.

Software-based interventions can be beneficial as they often have a level of artificial intelligence that adapts the program offered to the needs of the learner. For example, the program learns from the errors

Table 22.2 Features of intervention for dyslexia.

General features	Phonics based
	Explicit teaching of regular phonic patterns
	Additional teaching of irregular phonic exceptions and 'tricky' words, e.g. 'said'
	Working memory element
Examples	Fresh Start
	Rainbow Readers
	Alpha to Omega
	Lifeboat
	Toe by Toe
	Lexia
	Nessy Phonics
	Dyslexia Gold

Table 22.3 Features of intervention for dysgraphia.

General features	Use graphic organisers to support organisation and take away the fear of the empty page
	Enable editing
Examples	Write from the Start (pre-letter formation)
	Rainbow Writers
	Speech-to-text software such as DragonSpeak

Table 22.4 Features of intervention for dyscalculia.

General features	Based on understanding of basic number concepts
	Move from concrete to abstract concepts
	Make arithmetic learning a positive experience
	Avoid learning by rote
Examples	Number Shark
	Numicon
	Dienes Apparatus (Base 10 Equipment)
	Number Beads
	Dyslexia Gold

that the user makes and will present more examples and practice opportunities for the learner to ensure that the learning is embedded. Similarly, where the learner requires additional time to complete tasks, the program will slow down the rate at which it presents items.

Within the United Kingdom, the Education Endowment Foundation has produced a Teaching and Learning Toolkit that discusses the efficacy of different interventions and teaching approaches. It has also produced a guidance report on the use of teaching assistants (see Further Reading).

Assistive technology

Technology to support learners to access the wider curriculum has become much more refined in recent years.

Accessibility tools on laptops and tablets can enable the user to change the background colour on which text is presented. They can also read text to the user, and conversely the user can dictate what they want to write and have it appear as text.

Typing is a life skill that can support those who have difficulty with letter formation. The use of a spellchecker can also be helpful for those with spelling difficulties. These technologies can even be used in external examinations, where the use of a scribe might also be indicated as necessary.

Reading pens are available that read any printed text. These may be particularly useful in classes such as history, where the learner might be required to read long pieces of text, such as secondary source materials. They can be used in lieu of a reader in external examinations and have the added bonus of the learner being able to reread lines that they may not have understood.

Calculators are widely used, including in external examinations. However, the learner needs to be able to estimate whether an answer looks reasonable or not.

Voice recognition software has become more sophisticated. It requires frequent use to learn the user's specific speech patterns, but is beneficial and can replace a scribe in given circumstances.

Specialist teaching

A specialist teacher is a qualified teacher who has additional, postgraduate qualifications in dyslexia and learning difficulties, and has a current practising certificate. The interventions that are used by specialist teachers are highly structured, sequential phonics programmes, using multisensory activities with opportunities for over-learning. These are the hallmarks of any good phonics teaching or intervention, including those used within all mainstream schools.

Further reading

Butterworth, B. (2019). *Dyscalculia: From Science to Education*. London: Routledge.

Education Endowment Foundation (2015). Making best use of teaching assistants. https://educationendowmentfoundation.org.uk/education-evidence/guidance-reports/teaching-assistants

Education Endowment Foundation (2020). Teaching and Learning Toolkit. https://educationendowmentfoundation.org.uk/education-evidence/teaching-learning-toolkit

CHAPTER 23

Supporting Specific Learning Disorder into Adulthood

Tracy Laverick and Julie Armstrong

OVERVIEW

- The Equality Act 2010 legally protects anyone with a disability from discrimination and should ensure the use of reasonable adjustments to reduce the impact of a disability on their role.
- Modern technology, including the use of smartphones, computer accessibility programs and smart speakers, can aid aspects of a specific learning disorder.
- Individuals need to experiment with the technology that most supports them to overcome any barriers.

The rise in technology use has significantly aided adults who may have a specific learning disorder (SpLD), even at the severe end of the spectrum, with benefits for social and work use.

Equality Act 2010

The Equality Act 2010 defines a disability as 'a physical or mental impairment which has a substantial and long-term adverse effect on their ability to carry out normal day-to-day activities'. Substantial is defined as 'more than trivial'.

Therefore, individuals with an SpLD that has impacts on their normal day-to-day activities are covered under the Act and employers or educational institutions are required by law to make reasonable adjustments. These reasonable adjustments might include access to some of the technology described in this chapter. Employers and educational settings must ensure that individuals have access to the tools they require to perform to the best of their abilities and that they are not disadvantaged by their difficulties. Such adjustments must be put in place in collaboration with the individual.

Higher education

Each university will have a student support department where individuals can be advised on what is available. Students may require access arrangements, which might include additional time and computer use for exams. Marking of assignments can include leniency regarding word and sentence construction for students with identified SpLD, and tutors should be able to discuss this further with them. Within universities, students can use a range of accessibility settings on computers and may benefit from additional resources to do so.

Since Covid-19, it has become more possible to have lectures and meetings recorded so that they can be viewed again, at the individual's pace. Online meetings can be recorded 'within app' or using a smartphone so that main points are not missed. Everyone else in the meeting should be made fully aware if any session is recorded.

For many young adults, the move to the greater demands for reading at university may highlight their difficulties and although they may not have required additional support within their school years, they may require this for higher education.

Working on computers or other devices

The accessibility settings available on most computers and devices have improved immeasurably over the past few years. Speech to text can be used on most devices and has improved in its accuracy. Specific dictation programs can be used for more extensive writing requirements.

Accessibility settings allow for text, menus and web pages to be read out loud. The user may need to employ headphones in open working environments, but these can now be very discreet if required. Computer screens can be altered to have a lower contrast or to have a colour filter limiting the impact of visual stress.

Mobile phones, particularly smartphones, can store multiple reminders and alarms to aid memory and alleviate organisational difficulties that might be experienced. The increased use of smart speakers is helpful for this purpose, and speakers can be requested to complete basic functions such as spelling out words, computation and reading out information.

Instant access to the internet and calculators can aid the requirement for basic maths and the use of spreadsheets, supported by online video tutorials, can complete more complex calculations.

Leisure

Being able to enjoy books is now more accessible due to the large number of books and resources available as audio versions. A range of free and paid-for subscriptions can give access to most current literature.

E-books often allow for the text to be highlighted and read out, if the book is not available in an audio version.

Video is a common medium for information to be shared, whether this is for leisure or work purposes. Videos are not just for film and TV, but can explain how to acquire new skills or concepts and develop thinking.

Employment

None of the above measures completely ameliorates the difficulties experienced by an individual with an SpLD. All these activities will be more effortful and are likely to influence levels of fatigue and mental health and well-being. This can also be the reason why some individuals can be reticent to share knowledge about their difficulties with employers. As part of the Equality Act, employers and education providers should plan for SpLDs and how needs might be met even prior to an individual requiring this support. This normalises them within the workplace and therefore an employee with an SpLD is more likely to feel included.

The profile of needs for individuals is unique and employers and individuals should work collaboratively to identify the most effective package of support.

As part of the interview and application process, applicants should have the opportunity to share information regarding their SpLD so that reasonable adjustments can be made. For example, within the interview stage additional time to process answers may be required.

Further reading

British Dyslexia Association (n.d.). Advice for employers. https://www.bdadyslexia.org.uk/advice/employers

Office for Students (n.d.). Access agreements. https://www.officeforstudents.org.uk/advice-and-guidance/promoting-equal-opportunities/access-agreements

CHAPTER 24

Foetal Alcohol Spectrum Disorder

Elizabeth Birley

OVERVIEW

- Foetal alcohol spectrum disorder (FASD) can occur in persons exposed to alcohol in utero.

- There is no known safe limit of alcohol consumption in pregnancy. Even small amounts of alcohol may have a significant effect on the developing foetus.

- Alcohol is a neurotoxin. Exposure to alcohol in utero leads to changes in brain structure, size and functioning, as well as changes to other organs within the body.

- Abnormal development of the central nervous system is what leads to the neurodevelopmental profile seen in FASD.

- Reaching a diagnosis takes a multidisciplinary approach, using a multistep process.

- Once a diagnosis is confirmed, a holistic management plan needs to be formed covering all aspects of the young person's life.

- With the right support, children and young people with FASD can live long and fulfilling lives.

History and definitions

Foetal alcohol spectrum disorders (FASDs) occur in persons exposed to the neurotoxic effects of alcohol in utero. This is most commonly termed pre-natal alcohol exposure (PAE). As the name suggests, the nature of presenting complaints occurs along a spectrum.

Prior to the most recent evolution of diagnostic terms, a number of different diagnoses were used under the umbrella term of FASDs. Foetal alcohol syndrome (FAS) was thought to be at the most severe end of the spectrum, often having classical facial features, growth restriction and central nervous system (CNS) problems. Partial foetal alcohol syndrome (pFAS) was used when there was a history of maternal alcohol use in pregnancy and some, but not all, of the facial abnormalities as well as growth or CNS features. The diagnosis of alcohol-related neurodevelopmental disorder (ARND) was given to individuals who did not have abnormal facial features or growth restriction, but did display CNS features on a background of

PAE. Alcohol-related birth defects (ARBD) referred to abnormalities in how some organs were formed – heart, kidney, bones – in relation to PAE and could be used in conjunction with any of the other diagnostic terms (see Figure 24.1).

DSM-V-TR uses the equivalently termed neurobehavioural disorder associated with pre-natal alcohol exposure (ND-PAE). This is listed as a one of a number of 'conditions for further study' that may help inform future decisions about placement within the manual. Proposed diagnostic criteria for ND-PAE in individuals exposed to alcohol prenatally are noted. These include impairments in neurocognitive functioning, self-regulation and adaptive functioning, with an onset in childhood and without a better alternative diagnosis. Emphasis is given to how ND-PAE may be diagnosed in both the presence and absence of associated features, such as facial dysmorphology.

The Scottish Intercollegiate Guidelines Network (SIGN) produced the first UK clinical guideline for the recognition and diagnosis of FASD in 2019. The SIGN guidance has allowed UK clinicians to adopt a more standardised approach in diagnosing FASD by advocating for the simpler terms of FASD *with* sentinel facial features, FASD *without* sentinel facial features and those who are *at risk* of FASD. The SIGN156 guidance has now been incorporated into the National Institute for Health and Care Excellence (NICE) Quality Standard QS204 for FASD.

Epidemiology

The actual prevalence of FASD in the United Kingdom is unknown. The Department of Health and Social Care FASD health needs assessment 2021 identified a lack of robust prevalence estimates in England.

A 2017 study estimated the global prevalence of alcohol use in pregnancy at 9.8% and 41% in the United Kingdom. The study further estimated that 1 in every 67 women who consumed alcohol in pregnancy would deliver a child who would go on to be diagnosed with FAS.

An active case study performed in Greater Manchester in 2021 estimated a prevalence of FASD as between 1.8% and 3.6% of the population.

ABC of Neurodevelopmental Disorders, First Edition. Edited by Munib Haroon.
© 2024 John Wiley & Sons Ltd. Published 2024 by John Wiley & Sons Ltd.

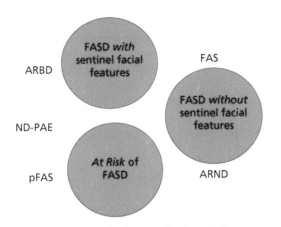

Figure 24.1 Descriptive terms for the neurodevelopmental consequences of pre-natal alcohol use past and present. The circled terms are those adopted by the UK guidance produced by the Scottish Intercollegiate Guidelines Network. ARBD, alcohol-related birth defects; ARND, alcohol-related neurodevelopmental disorder; FAS, foetal alcohol syndrome; FASD, foetal alcohol spectrum disorder; ND-PAE, neurobehavioural disorder associated with pre-natal alcohol exposure; pFAS, partial foetal alcohol syndrome.

Numerous studies have been performed in an attempt to estimate the prevalence of FASD in the population. All studies have their limitations; one limitation that is common to all is the sensitivity of the topic of PAE and the potential for reporting bias for alcohol use in pregnancy. Regardless of the exact number, it is reasonable to conclude that the actual prevalence of FASD is far higher than figures based on individuals presenting to services and receiving a formal diagnosis.

Aetiology

Alcohol is a known teratogen and there is no known safe limit of alcohol consumption in pregnancy. Identifying such limits remains challenging.

Alcohol is known to induce apoptosis. In a developing foetus, inappropriate apoptosis during organogenesis can lead to abnormal development of those organs. Abnormal development of the CNS is what leads to the neurodevelopmental profile seen in FASD. The CNS develops throughout pregnancy, and therefore exposure to alcohol at any stage in pregnancy can have an adverse impact on brain development and cause subsequent neurodevelopmental difficulties. In addition, alcohol also affects pre-conception, through epigenetic changes within male and female gametes, and the pregnancy itself. Women who drink alcohol during pregnancy are in general more likely to have poorer diets and more difficult lifestyles, such as exposure to domestic violence. These pregnancies are also at an increased risk of early miscarriage, premature delivery and placental insufficiency. These factors all confound the ability to understand the exact cause and effect, as it is not possible to study the effect of alcohol use in isolation.

Prevention

FASD seems relatively unique in the world of neurodevelopmental disorders in that it is an entirely preventable condition. Better awareness and understanding of the effects of alcohol during pregnancy are needed at a population level. Pre-conception abstention is the only way to be certain a pregnancy has not been affected by alcohol use, as even alcohol in early pregnancy, prior to a woman discovering that she is pregnant, has been shown to have adverse outcomes.

Diagnosis

Until fairly recently, understanding surrounding FASD was poor, with the majority of people believing that facial features needed to be present in order to make the diagnosis. In fact, FASD with facial features makes up a minority of the combined diagnoses.

The clinical presentation of FASD varies widely. Those children not identified in early childhood via risk, facial features and developmental impairment may progress through the earlier years of childhood without incident. It may not be until a child reaches secondary school, and academia becomes more challenging or difficult behaviours become more noticeable, that concerns may arise. Often, children with FASD may progress well within education up to a point, and then seem to begin to tail off in comparison to their peers. These children may then present to neurodevelopmental, community paediatric and Child and Adolescent Mental Health Services (CAMHS) clinics.

In order to make a clinical diagnosis a stepwise approach is required (see later in this chapter).

Assessing maternal alcohol use

It may seem obvious, but confirming the presence, or absence, of exposure to alcohol in utero is a key part of the diagnostic process. Due to the sensitivity of the issue, determining an accurate level of exposure is often challenging. In children who are looked after or adopted, information pertaining to the birth mother's alcohol consumption can be lost. Alcohol consumption in pregnancy may not be recorded in antenatal records, or if it is it may not be easily accessible to those not familiar with the obstetric records. Increasing awareness regarding FASD among health professionals is increasing the accuracy of how this information is recorded, but there is still a long way to go.

The first step in the diagnostic process involves categorising the children to one of three groups: PAE confirmed, PAE confirmed absent, PAE unknown. In order to confirm the presence or absence of alcohol use in pregnancy, an element of investigative work is often required. Sometimes there is clear evidence of severe alcohol dependence shortly after birth, but use during pregnancy may still be refuted. In this case reasonable judgement should be exercised based on the various sources of information available (Box 24.1).

As well as assessing if the mother used alcohol at all, it is important to determine at what level alcohol was used and at what point in the pregnancy. Various screening tools have been established for assessing alcohol use in the general population and one of these can be utilised.

If antenatal exposure to alcohol remains unknown, this has a substantial impact on the ability to offer a formal diagnosis. A diagnosis of FASD where PAE is unknown can only be made if all three sentinel facial features are present.

Box 24.1 **Sources of information when assessing PAE**

- Direct history from mother
- Witnessed by a reliable source, e.g. relative/child's guardian
- Evidence from antenatal visits or hospital birth records (appropriate consent must be sought to access these records)
- Evidence contained within social work or police files
- Clearly referenced evidence from looked-after or adoption medical reports

Assessing sentinel facial features

After PAE has been confirmed, or if it is still unknown, it is necessary then to assess the child for the sentinel facial features of FASD. The three sentinel features – smooth philtrum, thin upper lip and small palpebral fissures – have been found to be highly specific for FASD when found in combination. For this reason, in the presence of unknown PAE with all three sentinel facial features, a diagnosis of FASD may still be possible if the young person meets the neurodevelopmental criteria.

In the past, assessment of lip and philtrum has been highly subjective. Various standardised and validated tools for the assessment of facial features have been developed. Lip and philtrum appearance can be compared to pictorial guides, scoring the child's lip and philtrum separately. Centile charts have also been produced for the measurement of palpebral fissure (PF) length. The PF length should be measured from the inner canthus to the outer canthus (the extremities of the eyelid) as accurately as possible using a clear ruler and then plotted on the chart. A PF length of >2 standard deviations (SD) below the mean for age would be a positive result (see Figure 24.2).

Despite attempts to standardise the assessment of facial features, it remains subjective. Photographic analysis software has become fairly commonplace and more advanced 3D technologies are also in development.

Other dysmorphic features have been described in individuals with FASD: ptosis of the eyelids, epicanthal folds, strabismus and 'rail road track' ears. None of these features is required to make the diagnosis.

Assessing neurodevelopmental impairment

The neurodevelopmental presentation of FASD has many overlapping features with other neurodevelopmental conditions. Without confirmed PAE or sentinel facial features, it would be impossible to attribute the neurodevelopmental difficulties to PAE due to the vast amount of other possible underlying factors. According to SIGN, 10 areas of potential neurodevelopmental impairment are assessed when considering a diagnosis of FASD (see Table 24.1).

Table 24.1 The 10 areas of neurodevelopmental assessment.

Brain structure	Microcephaly (occipitofrontal circumference of <3rd centile)
	Seizure disorders
	Structural brain abnormalities, e.g. agenesis of the corpus callosum.
Motor skills	Fine motor skills: manual dexterity, handwriting
	Gross motor skills: balance, coordination
Cognition	Intelligence quotient (IQ)
	Working memory
	Verbal and non-verbal reasoning
	Processing speeds
Language	Expressive language
	Receptive language
Academic achievement	Reading
	Literacy
	Numeracy
Memory	Verbal
	Visual
Attention	Concentration
	Task focus and distractibility
	Organisational skills
Executive functioning	Higher-level thinking skills
	Impulse control
	Hyperactivity
Affect regulation	Mood disorders, depression
	Anxiety disorder: generalised anxiety disorder, phobias, obsessive compulsive disorder, panic disorder
	Conduct disorder
	Oppositional defiant disorder
Adaptive behaviour	Social skills: interpersonal relationships, empathy, ability to form friendships
	Practical skills: activities of daily living, money management, personal care
	Social communication

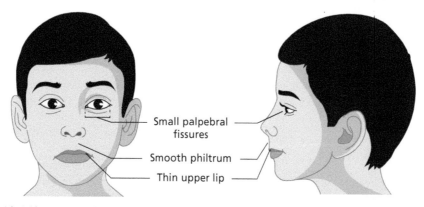

Small palpebral fissures

Smooth philtrum

Thin upper lip

Figure 24.2 All three sentinel facial features must be present for a diagnosis of foetal alcohol spectrum disorder with sentinel facial features.

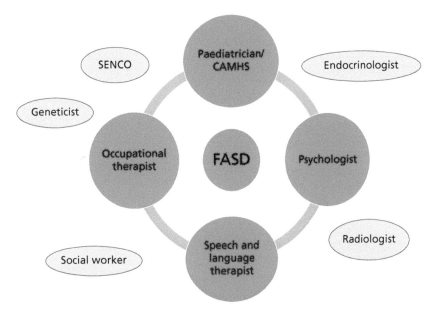

Figure 24.3 Professionals involved in multidisciplinary assessment of a young person with foetal alcohol spectrum disorder (FASD). CAMHS, Child and Adolescent Mental Health Services; SENCO, special educational needs coordinator.

Full assessment of the neurodevelopmental areas requires a multidisciplinary approach, and often involves access to standardised testing to confirm impairment within each area (see Figure 24.3). The assessment process will vary significantly, depending on local provision and access to appropriate specialist input. Where local services are not adequately equipped to assess children and young people for FASD, referrals can be made to larger regional and national services, though this may require additional funding to be secured.

Where a child with all three sentinel facial features is too young to engage in a meaningful developmental assessment, diagnosis of FASD with sentinel facial features may still be given in the presence of microcephaly. It would remain important to undertake a thorough neurodevelopmental assessment at the point it becomes appropriate to do so.

Assessment of growth and other associated features

Historically, growth retardation has been included among the diagnostic criteria for FASD. More recently it has been found that FASD can exist without a child having an impairment in growth. However, there is still a recognised association with growth impairment and FASD. Any child under assessment for FASD should have their height, weight and head circumference measured regularly and plotted on the appropriate growth chart. Any concerns should be thoroughly assessed, with referral on to endocrine services as necessary.

In addition to growth impairment, various other physical associations have been noted including, but not limited to, renal abnormalities, musculoskeletal problems and disordered metabolism. FASD is a full-systems condition and a holistic approach to assessment should always be encouraged.

Assessment of other possible causes of presentation

An important but often overlooked aspect of the diagnostic process for FASD is the assessment of other possible causes of the child's presenting difficulties; these children have frequently had difficult and traumatic backgrounds. They may have been exposed to other substances in utero, have experienced developmental trauma and been exposed to adverse childhood experiences. They may be suffering from disordered attachment or other types of psychological difficulties related to their backgrounds. All of these must be assessed and the impact considered when formulating a diagnosis.

Another important factor is if there are any underlying genetic abnormalities that may also account for the presenting difficulties. Many agencies will state the importance of ruling out genetic factors prior to making a diagnosis of FASD. Genetic abnormalities must always be considered and discussed as part of the multidisciplinary team assessment. However, within the fast-paced field of clinical genetics available tests and eligibility criteria are always evolving. A good understanding of local pathways and a relationship with clinical geneticist colleagues is invaluable.

An approach to assessment and diagnosis is shown in Box 24.2 and Table 24.2.

Management

Due to the wide and varied difficulties of young people with FASD, there is no 'one size fits all' approach to management. Ongoing follow-up and management could be led by a number of different professionals depending on the child's needs; a collaborative approach is paramount (see Figure 24.4). A young person with comorbid psychiatric diagnoses may benefit from a psychiatrist

Box 24.2 **Approach to child presenting with possible FASD**

- *Does the child have neurodevelopmental impairment?* If yes, take a full neurodevelopmental history, including exploration of possible other causes.
- *Is there a reliable history of alcohol use in pregnancy?* If no, is it possible to acquire information from other sources?
- *Does the child have all three sentinel facial features of FASD?* If not, and there is not a reliable history of PAE, consider other diagnoses.
- *Does the child have microcephaly?* Diagnoses may be given in young children with confirmed alcohol exposure, all three sentinel facial features and microcephaly, prior to full neurodevelopmental assessment.
- *Is the child of an appropriate age to have a meaningful neurodevelopmental assessment?* Consider which areas of neurodevelopment are a cause for concern. Consider which professionals will be required and what local provision is available to undertake further assessment.
- *Does the child have an impairment in three areas of neurodevelopment?* An impairment in 3 of the 10 areas of neurodevelopment is required to reach a diagnosis in school-aged children with or without sentinel facial features.
- *Is there any growth impairment?* Consider further investigations or referrals as required (e.g. blood tests, dietician, endocrinology).
- *Are there any other associated features?* Consider further investigation or onward referral as required.
- *Is the family well supported?* Check the support network. Signpost to resources, parent groups, etc. Make onward referrals as needed (e.g. health visitor, early years support, early help).

Table 24.2 Diagnostic algorithm based on Sign156 guidance.

Pre-school-aged child (aged <6yr) Confirmed PAE?	All three sentinel facial features?	Microcephaly?	Diagnosis
PAE confirmed absent	N/A	N/A	No FASD diagnosis
Unknown	No	N/A	
	Yes	Yes	FASD *with* sentinel facial features
		No	*At risk* of FASD
Yes	No	No	
		Yes	
	Yes	No	
		Yes	FASD *with* sentinel facial features

School-aged child (aged >6yr) Confirmed PAE?	All three sentinel facial features?	Three areas of impairment on neurodevelopmental assessment?	Diagnosis
PAE confirmed absent	N/A	N/A	No FASD diagnosis
Unknown	No	N/A	
	Yes	No	
		Yes	FASD *with* sentinel facial features
Yes	Yes	Yes	FASD *with* sentinel facial features
		No	*At risk* of FASD
	No	No	
		Yes	FASD *without* sentinel facial features

FASD, foetal alcohol spectrum disorder; N/A, not applicable; PAE, pre-natal alcohol exposure. *Source:* Adapted from Scottish Intercollegiate Guidelines Network (2019).

taking the lead role in their care. Equally, a young person whose main difficulties revolve around learning impairment may be better coordinated by educational professionals. Contributing to the young person's management plan is a key part of a clinician's role when working with young people with FASD, even if the ongoing follow-up is not directly led by that person.

Support and advocacy

Children with FASD can reside in many families, including birth families. However, the high number of young people with FASD being raised in foster or adoptive families goes some way to demonstrate the complex needs of children and young people with FASD. Families can often be tired, overwhelmed, frustrated and sleep deprived, among many other things. Due to the challenges of caring for a child with FASD, sadly these children are often at risk of placement breakdown and multiple foster placements. Children living with birth families are often exposed to open discrimination due to lack of understanding from the general public. Educating parents and carers about FASD and signposting to local services and support groups is one of the most important aspects of management. In addition, as children get older, peer support and a feeling of 'belonging' can have the most profound effect on outcomes. Clinicians are ideally placed to signpost young people and carers to local and national support networks and to advocate for patients within education, health and social care as required.

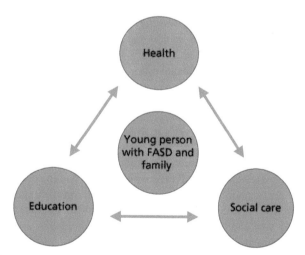

Figure 24.4 Management requires a collaborative approach between all those involved in the life of a young person with foetal alcohol spectrum disorder (FASD).

Physical and mental health

Often assessment and management of individual aspects can make a huge difference to a young person's quality of life, for example sleep disturbance or sensory processing difficulties. Behavioural problems are frequently reported and individual approaches to behavioural management can be hugely successful, when correctly understood by the young person's support network.

Management of any individual areas of identified neurodevelopmental impairment is typically the cornerstone of ongoing management plans, such as speech and language therapy or occupational therapy.

Additional diagnoses, for example of attention deficit hyperactivity disorder (ADHD), should be managed accordingly by the use of appropriate medications, therapies and interventions by the relevant specialists.

However associated features are managed, it is important that young people are continually assessed following diagnosis. New features may emerge through time requiring amended or entirely different approaches. Continued and repeated assessment will be required, particularly at key transition points.

Education

Supporting children and young people within education can be one of the most challenging elements of management. Due to the varied needs of children with FASD, they can attend any number of different educational settings, from mainstream school with little additional informal support, to special educational needs settings with Education, Health and Care plans (EHCPs). It is important that the school or educational setting is a key contributor in the development and implementation of any management plans. All aspects of the educational environment need to be considered. Environments should be assessed for suitability and transition periods should be anticipated and planned for. Appropriate training regarding FASD and its multifaceted presentations should be provided for all educational professionals involved with the young person. Educational psychologists can be key people within a child's care plan and should be utilised at every opportunity. Most importantly, a close working relationship between families and education is paramount to a young person's success within education.

Transition to adulthood

As with all conditions, transition planning needs to be considered and addressed early. Once a young person reaches the age of 18, paediatric services and the associated support available within those services will often be closed to them. At the time of writing, specific services for adults with FASD are few and far between, if they exist at all. As the condition becomes more recognised and the far-reaching effects better understood, this may improve. In the meantime, transition to adult services needs to be carefully considered and planned.

Repeat assessment of neurodevelopmental impairment would be beneficial, with identification of any adult services able to address any difficulties identified. Another important consideration is the young person's understanding and whether or not they can be deemed to have adequate capacity. Depending on the child's individual circumstances, disability social workers or advocates may be required.

An important consideration is those young people residing in foster care. Once a young person turns 18, they will leave care. Appropriate plans need to be in place for these young people to ensure they have appropriate support in line with their own individual abilities and needs. Children who reside with birth parents and who also have additional learning or neurodevelopmental needs may continue to be supported by their families throughout their adult life. Sadly, due to the high proportion of young people with FASD cared for by the local authorities, this may not be the case for a large number of children and young people with FASD. Clear and effective communication between health and social care colleagues is often key in the lifelong management of these individuals (Figure 24.4).

Prognosis and outcome

Often children undergoing assessment for FASD receive multiple additional diagnoses. including autism spectrum disorder (ASD), ADHD and intellectual disability. There is an association with mental health difficulties and suicide – with rates increasing through late adolescence and early adulthood. There is also an association with an increased risk for later tobacco, alcohol and other substance use.

Despite the overlap of presentations within each diagnosis, it is important to note that FASD is irreparable brain damage caused by the mother's ingestion of a teratogenic substance during pregnancy. For this reason, FASD may not always be considered as a neurodevelopmental disorder, though it has neurodevelopmental consequences. This can be an important distinction, as not only is it relevant to understand any underlying cause of a given diagnosis, but this particular issue can be a sensitive one among parents and carers within the neurodiverse community.

If FASD is not recognised, diagnosed and appropriately managed, these children and young people can be labelled as 'naughty', a label that tends to stick and may additionally contribute to poorer health, educational and social outcomes. Knowing about FASD and receiving a diagnosis are key to understanding how to access support. FASD is a life-long condition. It does not get better; children do not 'grow out' of it. That said, presenting features can change over time. With appropriate support and management of associated difficulties, children and young people can live long and fulfilling lives into adulthood.

Further reading

American Psychiatric Association (2023). *Diagnostic and Statistical Manual of Mental Disorders*, 5e. Text Revision. Washington, DC: American Psychiatric Publishing.

Astley, S.J. (2004). *Diagnostic Guide for Fetal Alcohol Spectrum Disorders: The 4-Digit Diagnostic Code*. Seattle, WA: University of Washington.

Brown, J.M., Bland, R., Jonsson, E., and Greenshaw, A.J. (2019). A brief history of awareness of the link between alcohol and fetal alcohol spectrum disorder. *Canadian Journal of Psychiatry* 64 (3): 164–168.

Department of Health and Social Care. (2021). Fetal alcohol spectrum disorder: health needs assessment. https://www.gov.uk/government/publications/fetal-alcohol-spectrum-disorder-health-needs-assessment/fetal-alcohol-spectrum-disorder-health-needs-assessment

McCarthy, R., Mukherjee, R.A., Fleming, K.M. et al. (2021). Prevalence of fetal alcohol spectrum disorder in Greater Manchester, UK: an active case ascertainment study. *Alcoholism: Clinical and Experimental Research* 45 (11): 2271–2281.

Mukherjee, R.A. and Aiton, N. (ed.) (2021). *Prevention, Recognition and Management of Fetal Alcohol Spectrum Disorders*. New York: Springer International.

National Institute of Health and Care Excellence (NICE) (2022). Fetal alcohol spectrum disorder. Quality standard [QS204]. https://www.nice.org.uk/guidance/qs204

National Organisation for FASD (2022). The time is now: the national perspective on ramping up FASD prevention, diagnosis and support services. https://nationalfasd.org.uk/wp-content/uploads/2022/03/National-FASD-RT-Report-v004-INTERACTIVE-singles-2.pdf

Popova, S., Lange, S., Probst, C. et al. (2017). Estimation of national, regional, and global prevalence of alcohol use during pregnancy and fetal alcohol syndrome: a systematic review and meta-analysis. *Lancet Global Health* 5 (3): e290–e299.

Scottish Intercollegiate Guidelines Network (SIGN) (2019). SIGN156: Children and young people exposed prenatally to alcohol. http://www.sign.ac.uk/media/1092/sign156.pdf

Surrey and Borders Partnership NHS Foundation Trust (n.d.). National Clinic for Fetal Alcohol Spectrum Disorders. www.fasdclinic.com.

CHAPTER 25

Mental Health Conditions in Children and Young People with Neurodevelopmental Disorders

Monica Shaha, Mini Pillay, and Munib Haroon

> **OVERVIEW**
>
> - Individuals with neurodevelopmental disorders (NDDs) are at increased risk of mental health difficulties.
> - Anxiety is the commonest psychiatric comorbidity in NDDs.
> - The high prevalence of psychiatric comorbidity needs to be taken into account when planning mental health and neurodevelopmental services.
> - When assessing a child or young person with an NDD, the possibility of a coexisting mental health condition should always be borne in mind.

Neurodevelopmental disorders (NDDs) include a wide range of conditions. As a principle, while all NDD's are associated with a higher risk of mental health difficulties, the following three chapters will focus on some of the difficulties encountered in:
- Autism spectrum disorder
- Attention deficit hyperactivity disorder (ADHD)
- Tic disorders

In these conditions, important comorbid mental health conditions can include:
- Anxiety disorders
- Depressive disorders
- Obsessive compulsive disorder (OCD) and related conditions
- Schizophrenia spectrum and other psychotic disorders
- Feeding and eating disorders
- Oppositional defiant disorder (ODD) and conduct disorder (particularly important to consider in ADHD and tic disorders)

Anxiety disorders

Anxiety is a normal response to an unusual or stressful event, and can be seen as the psychological component of the 'flight or fight' response. Anxiety is considered abnormal when:
- It is excessively severe or prolonged
- It occurs in the absence of a stressful event
- It impairs social, physical or occupational functioning

There are several types of anxiety disorders, including generalised anxiety disorder, panic disorder, social anxiety disorder and various phobia-related disorders.

Depressive disorders

Depression is a mood disorder in which the predominant feelings are of sadness, hopelessness and emptiness. This may be accompanied by changes in a person's ability to carry out day-to-day activities or to function normally. This may be noted as a loss of interest or pleasure in activities, weight loss, abnormal sleeping patterns, abnormal psychomotor symptoms, reduced energy, feelings of worthlessness, reduced focus or indecisiveness and recurrent thoughts of death or suicidal ideation. A depressive episode may be part of a lifetime pattern of mood disorder.

Obsessive compulsive disorder

OCD is characterised by the presence of obsessions and/or compulsions. Obsessions are recurrent and persistent thoughts, urges or mental images that cause anxiety because of their intrusive and unpleasant nature. Compulsions are repetitive behaviours or mental acts that a person with OCD feels the urge to do in response to an obsessive thought or according to a rule that must be rigidly applied. These symptoms can interfere with all aspects of life, such as work, school and personal relationships.

Schizophrenia spectrum and other psychotic disorders

The features of these disorders include delusions (fixed beliefs not amenable to change when presented with conflicting evidence), hallucinations (perceptual experiences that have no external stimulus, e.g. seeing or hearing things that others do not see or hear), disorganised thinking and speech, disorganised or abnormal motor behaviour, and negative symptoms such as diminished emotional expression, avolition (diminished purposeful activities that are self-initiated), reduced speech (alogia), reduced social interaction

ABC of Neurodevelopmental Disorders, First Edition. Edited by Munib Haroon.
© 2024 John Wiley & Sons Ltd. Published 2024 by John Wiley & Sons Ltd.

(asociality) and a reduced ability to experience pleasure (anhedonia). These symptoms, or a resemblance to them, can also appear in some other mental health conditions or be suggestive of organic conditions such as Alzheimer's disease or brain tumours; they may also be a feature of a substance-induced psychotic disorder.

Feeding and eating disorders

The characteristic features of such disorders are disturbances in eating behaviours and related thoughts and emotions, which lead to altered food consumption/absorption and can then impair physical, emotional or mental health. Eating disorders can be serious and potentially fatal illnesses. Familiar eating disorders include anorexia nervosa, bulimia nervosa and binge-eating disorder. Other eating disorders that can appear in children include pica (eating non-nutritive, non-food substances on a persistent basis) and avoidant restrictive food intake disorder (an avoidance or lack of interest in food, which is associated with weight loss, nutritional deficiency, dependence on supplements or enteral feeds, and psychosocial dysfunctioning).

Oppositional defiant disorder

All children are oppositional from time to time, particularly when tired, hungry, stressed or upset. They may argue, talk back, disobey and defy parents, teachers and other adults. Oppositional behaviour is a normal part of development for 2–3-year-olds and early adolescents. However, openly uncooperative and hostile behaviour becomes a serious concern when it is so frequent and consistent that it stands out when compared with other children of the same age and developmental level and when it affects the child's social, family and academic life.

In children with ODD, there is an ongoing pattern of behaviour (by definition episodes should occur more than weekly for >6 months in those over 5 years of age). It is characterised by anger/irritable mood, argumentative/defiant behaviour (which may be towards other children – and not just siblings – adults, authority figures and rules) and vindictiveness. The features cause distress to the individual or others in their lives (home, school, social) and have a negative impact in/on these settings.

Conduct disorder

'Conduct disorder' refers to a group of repetitive and persistent behavioural and emotional problems in youngsters. Children and adolescents with this disorder have great difficulty following rules, respecting the rights of others, showing empathy and behaving in a socially acceptable way. This may manifest as aggression to people and animals, destruction of property (including deliberate fire setting), deceitfulness, lying, stealing and serious violations of rules.

Comorbidity in individual neurodevelopmental disorders

Although it can be useful to quote prevalence estimates, it is important to state that these are estimates and that prevalence will vary according to underlying differences in the chosen population and inclusion/exclusion criteria (for example those based on age, sex and the presence/absence of other comorbidities) and the mode of ascertaining individual diagnoses. Although Chapters 25–27 focus on three conditions, it is important to remember that mental health difficulties are observed in all neurodevelopmental disorders (see Box 25.1).

Autism spectrum disorder

There is an increased prevalence of different psychiatric disorders in autistic people (Tables 25.1 and 25.2). It is important to note that these figures will vary according to the population being assessed, inclusion/exclusion criteria and what is classed as a psychiatric condition/disorder (for example, ADHD is included as a psychiatric disorder in many studies).

Box 25.1 **Specific learning difficulties, developmental coordination disorder, intellectual development disorder and mental health**

Compared to children without, children with specific learning difficulties are at a moderately increased risk of experiencing the symptoms of anxiety or depression, as well as externalising symptoms like aggression. The exact reasons for this are poorly understood and it may be that particular sub-groups are more at risk – for example, those with other comorbidities. It is likely that there are other risk factors and protective factors that may modify the likelihood of these symptoms escalating into a diagnosed disorder, such as the presence of supportive family, friends and teachers, as well a child's own coping strategies and resilience. This remains an area of ongoing inquiry.

Children with developmental coordination disorder (DCD) are at an increased risk of mental health issues. Theoretically this could be due in part to the presence of comorbidities, such as ADHD, and a degree of shared underlying genetic risk, where particular genes increase the expression of different phenotypes (pleiotropy), such as DCD and mental health difficulties. However, evidence also suggests that the presence of motor coordination problems has impacts on a child's social development, for example by limiting the games and sports they can partake in, leading to them becoming socially isolated; it can have a knock-on effect on self-esteem and maybe increase the risk of them being targeted for abuse by bullies, all of which can increase the risk of mental health issues. Once again, having a strong supportive network of peers and adults may play a protective role.

Children with intellectual development disorder (IDD) are at increased risk of developing mental health issues and almost 40–50% of them may present with recognisable symptoms of a mental health disorder. There are a number of challenges in identifying these disorders, including communication difficulties that can be present in IDD and diagnostic overshadowing, where professionals attribute the symptoms of a mental health disorder to the pre-existing neurodevelopmental condition.

Table 25.1 Prevalence of psychiatric disorders among individuals with autism compared to the general population (approximate figures).

Psychiatric disorder	General population (%)	Autistic population (%)
Any mental health disorder	20	80
Anxiety disorders	10	40
Depressive disorders	5	11–26
Schizophrenia spectrum and other psychotic disorders	1	3
Obsessive compulsive disorder	<2	9–17

Table 25.2 Eating disorders and the association with autism (approximate figures).

Feeding and eating disorder	Comparative data
All eating disorders	20–30% of adults with eating disorders are autistic 3–10% of children and young people with eating disorders are autistic
Pica	3.5% of children in the general population have pica 28.1% of children with autism and a co-occurring intellectual disability and 14% of children with autism but no intellectual disability have pica
Anorexia nervosa	Lifetime prevalence of up to 4% among females, 0.3% among males, in the general population Around 20% of women being treated for anorexia may be autistic

Attention deficit hyperactivity disorder

As has been noted in Chapters 2–5, alongside the core traits of hyperactivity, impulsivity and inattention, ADHD can be associated with a range of emotional and behaviour issues. In addition, there is a strong association with a number of mental health conditions. This may be because of pleiotropic genetic effects, but it may also be that the long-term burden of dealing with ADHD can lead to these conditions. For example, the restlessness that can be so characteristic of ADHD can often blur into feelings of being 'on edge'. These may tip the person over into being anxious, while the consequences of ADHD, which may include difficult social and familial relations and falling behind academically, may lead to children and adolescents developing mood-related issues.

The prevalence rates for different mental health conditions will vary according to underlying differences in the chosen population and inclusion/exclusion criteria (for example, based on age, sex and the presence/absence of other comorbidities) and the mode of ascertaining individual diagnoses, but suggested estimates for mental health disorders in paediatric/adolescent ADHD have included ~50% for conduct disorders, ~33% for mood disorders and 25–50% for anxiety disorders.

Tic disorders

Tourette's syndrome is frequently comorbid with other psychiatric conditions, such as OCD, depression, anxiety disorder or self-injurious behaviours, as well as medical conditions such as sleep disorders and migraines. About 85–88% of patients with Tourette's

syndrome have at least one comorbidity that usually appears between the ages of 4 and 10 years. The most common comorbidities are ADHD (average prevalence 50–60%) and OCD (average lifetime prevalence 30–50%). Other disorders (e.g. mood disorder, anxiety, disruptive behaviour, self-injurious behaviour) have been found to occur in about 30% of patients. About 10% of young people with tic disorders experience suicidal thoughts and attempts, which often occur in the context of anger, frustration and low mood.

Eating disorders such as anorexia nervosa and bulimia nervosa are present in 2% of patients with Tourette's syndrome; there is a female predominance and an onset in adolescence (15–19 years old). Disruptive behaviours and rage episodes, including explosive anger, temper outbursts, irritability and aggressiveness, are reported in 25–70% of Tourette's syndrome patients. ODD is reported in approximately 11–54% of Tourette's syndrome patients and conduct disorder in approximately 6–20%.

Conclusion

There is a high incidence of comorbid psychiatric disorders in NDDs. This needs to be taken into consideration when planning and delivering mental health and neurodevelopmental services. When assessing children with neurodevelopmental conditions, the possibility of mental health issues being present should always be borne in mind, and where a patient has difficulty in expressing their feelings and emotions, additional care should be taken before ruling out their presence.

Further reading

American Psychiatric Association (2022). *Diagnostic and Statistical Manual of Mental Health Disorders*, 5e. Text Revision. Washington, DC: American Psychiatric Association.

Barkley, R.A. (2018). *Attention Deficit Hyperactivity Disorder*. New York: Guilford Press.

Buckley, B., Glasson, E.J., Chen, W. et al. (2020). Prevalence estimates of mental health problems in children and adolescents with intellectual disability: a systematic review and meta-analysis. *Australian and New Zealand Journal of Psychiatry* 54 (10): 970–984. https://doi.org/10.1177/0004867420924101.

Fields, V.L. and Soke, G.N. (2021). Pica, autism and other disabilities. *Pediatrics* 147 (2): e20200462. https://doi.org/10.1542/peds.2020-0462.

Harrowell, I., Hollén, L., Lingam, R., and Emond, A. (2017). Mental health outcomes of developmental coordination disorder in late adolescence. *Developmental Medicine and Child Neurology* 59 (9): 973–979. https://doi.org/10.1111/dmcn.13469.

Lai, M.C., Kassee, C., Besney, R. et al. (2019). Prevalence of co-occurring mental health diagnoses in the autism population: a systematic review and meta-analysis. *Lancet Psychiatry* 6 (10): 819–829. https://doi.org/10.1016/S2215-0366(19)30289-5.

Meier, S.M., Petersen, L., Schendel, D.L. et al. (2015). Obsessive-compulsive disorder and autism spectrum disorders: longitudinal and offspring risk. *PLoS One* 10 (11): e0141703.

Rodgers, J. and Ofield, A. (2018). Understanding, recognising and treating co-occuring anxiety in autism. *Current Developmental Disorders Reports* 5: 58–64.

Ueda, K. and Black, K.J. (2021). A comprehensive review of tic disorders in children. *Journal of Clinical Medicine* 10 (11): 2479.

Wilmot, A., Hasking, P. et al. (2023). Understanding mental health in developmental dyslexia: a scoping review. *International Journal of Environmental Research and Public Health* 20 (2): 1653. https://doi.org/10.3390/ijerph20021653.

CHAPTER 26

Assessing Mental Health Conditions in Children and Young People with Neurodevelopmental Disorders

Monica Shaha and Mini Pillay

OVERVIEW

- A mental health diagnosis can provide an explanation and a route for further treatment and support.
- Remember to think about the possibility of medical conditions that could explain a change in a child's presentation.

Why is a diagnosis important?

As well as providing an explanation for a patient's clinical presentation (to the patient, family/carers and teachers), a psychiatric diagnosis can act as a gateway for further support and other services like certain types of therapy and medication. While the absence of a diagnosis should not be a barrier to gaining support at school, a diagnosis can help with clarifying exactly what is going on and what is required (Figure 26.1).

Making a diagnosis

A psychiatric diagnosis is made when all criteria for a particular condition are met. This commonly includes:
- Meeting a defined set/number of symptoms
- Having had symptoms for six months
- Psychosocial dysfunction – symptoms must impact on a child's ability to attend school, see friends, engage in usual activities of daily living and cause significant distress to the child
- The symptoms are not attributable to other mental disorders – meeting this criterion commonly lends itself to differences in opinion between clinicians, and decisions commonly come down to what is in child's best interests (to diagnose or not)

Screening tools or diagnostic questionnaires

There are many validated questionnaires for use in children:
- Generic screening tools for anxiety, depression, obsessive compulsive disorder (OCD), panic and separation anxiety – e.g. Revised Child Anxiety and Depression Scale (RCADS) for child/parent

- To gauge a child's overall functioning and the impact symptoms have on functioning – Strengths and Difficulties Questionnaire (SDQ) for self/parent/teacher
- For eating disorders – SCOFF, Eating Disorder Examination Questionnaire (EDE-Q)
- For OCD – Obsessive-Compulsive Inventory (OCI), Obsessional Compulsive Inventory (ChOCI)
- For psychosis – Positive and Negative Syndrome Scale (PANSS)

RCADS and SDQ are commonly used in multiple settings. The latter three are more typically used within Child and Adolescent Mental Health Services (CAMHS). None of the above tools should be used in isolation, as they are not diagnostic questionnaires. They can however serve two key purposes:
- As a baseline for a child's mental health
- In gauging response to treatment, whether that be from medication or therapy, or both

How to talk to children to elicit psychological/psychiatric symptoms

It can be tricky for children to open up about their struggles, perhaps more so if they have associated neurodevelopmental disorders (NDDs). Box 26.1 highlights a few key points to help these children to feel at ease.

Taking a psychiatric history and conducting a mental state examination

This is a crucial part of the diagnosis and takes the following format:
- Presenting complaint/history of presenting complaint – the concerns that have made the parent/child seek help. Ask about duration, what remediation has been tried and whether it has helped. Ask about mood, sleep patterns, appetite, energy levels, concentration, worries/anxieties, self-esteem, hobbies/interests. For more complex experiences, e.g. eliciting psychotic symptoms (see Box 26.2), it can help to ask: 'Have you ever had any strange experiences, for example have you ever seen or heard things that aren't there and that other people can't see or hear?'

ABC of Neurodevelopmental Disorders, First Edition. Edited by Munib Haroon.
© 2024 John Wiley & Sons Ltd. Published 2024 by John Wiley & Sons Ltd.

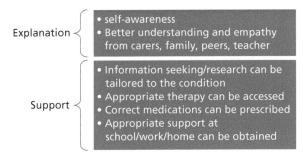

Explanation
- self-awareness
- Better understanding and empathy from carers, family, peers, teacher

Support
- Information seeking/research can be tailored to the condition
- Appropriate therapy can be accessed
- Correct medications can be prescribed
- Appropriate support at school/work/home can be obtained

Figure 26.1 Why a diagnosis is important.

Box 26.1 **How to Talk to Children and Young People at Clinic**

Find a quiet time and space to chat
  Start with a general question, for example 'How are you doing?'
  Pick up on cues they may share, for example 'You just mentioned you're struggling to fall asleep – shall we chat more about this?'
  Listen to what children say, offer comfort and validate their feelings

---

Box 26.2 **Assessing Possible Psychotic Experiences in Children**

Possible psychotic symptoms may include:
- Hearing noises/voices – children with NDDs frequently experience hearing noises/voices; however, these are rarely a symptom of an underlying psychotic illness. If a child tells you they hear the noises/voices with their ears, it can be helpful to ask, 'How do you hear the noises, with your ear, like you're hearing me talk to you right now?' It can also be helpful to ask, 'Do the noises sound like they're coming from inside your head?' Further screening for possible psychosis may be required. Using tools, for example PANSS, can also help.
- Seeing things – this can also be a common experience for children with NDDs. Typically, differentiating between possible psychotic/non-psychotic symptoms requires exploration of how they see the image, for example: 'Is it like it is in the corner of your eye?', 'If you look directly at it, does it disappear?' or 'When you look at it does it remain quite clear?'

- Past medical history – including any medical conditions, any prescribed medications, any allergies
- Drug history – including the use of alcohol, drugs, smoking status
- Past psychiatric history – any previous contact with CAMHS, private services
- Family history – ask about who is important to the child. Are there any psychiatric diagnoses in the extended family? (This is important, as the likelihood of a psychiatric diagnosis is higher in a child if a first-degree relative has the same diagnosis)
- Developmental history – ask about milestones. Enquiring about aspects to do with childhood socialisation and communication may be especially important if autism is suspected.
- Mental state examination – assess how the child presents, including their appearance and behaviour, their mood, their speech,

their thought processes (including risk to self/others), perceptual abnormalities, general cognition and insight into their current struggles

Assessing possible psychotic or unusual symptoms

Children with NDDs frequently experience what some may believe are psychotic symptoms (Box 26.2). However, further exploration of the experiences generally elucidates the character and phenomenology.

Children with NDDs may also experience unusual tastes or smells. It is important to take these seriously, as they may represent a possible underlying physical health condition, such as temporal lobe epilepsy.

Diagnostic overshadowing and neurodevelopmental disorders

The concept of diagnostic overshadowing refers to mistakenly attributing symptoms to a known/likely diagnosis as opposed to considering alternative explanations. The case study in Box 26.3 highlights the possibility of associated mental health diagnoses.

In clinical practice, presumed comorbid symptoms in children with NDDs, like attention deficit hyperactivity disorder (ADHD), for example suspected anxiety, frequently dissipate once the ADHD is treated.

When to refer to child and adolescent mental health services

In the United Kingdom, a lot of work around the management of mental health issues occurs prior to intervention by CAMHS. In England, the National Institute for Health and Care Excellence (NICE) has recommendations on when to refer children

---

Box 26.3 **Cody**

Cody is a 12-year-old boy with a known diagnosis of ADHD and autism spectrum disorder. He has a six-month history of emotional dysregulation, sleep-onset difficulty, restricted diet and loss of interest in playing with Lego, with some recent attempts to hurt himself by banging his head against the wall. During initial assessment, Cody is generally fit and well. He takes methylphenidate immediate release 10 mg twice daily for his attentional difficulties associated with his ADHD diagnosis.
  Possible differential diagnoses to consider might be:
- Mood symptoms secondary to methylphenidate prescription
- An emergent comorbid depressive disorder
- Difficulties due to associated physical health issues

  Differentiating between the first two requires investigating whether there is a temporal relationship between the use of stimulant medication and the onset of mood symptoms (or determining that the mood symptoms pre-date the medication). In this case, it is also important to consider assessing the risk of head banging as a self-harming behaviour (see later discussion).

presenting with mental health difficulties to secondary care. For example:

- In depression, referral should occur if there are two or more other risk factors for depression, or where one or more family members have multiple risk histories for depression
- In mild depression, referral should follow in those who have not responded to interventions in tier 1 after 2–3 months
- In more severe or recurrent forms of depression, a referral should happen in the face of ongoing self-neglect (>1 month) or if accompanied by active suicidal ideation/planning or where it is requested by carers or the patient

However, with services being stretched to the limit following the Covid-19 pandemic, the likelihood that all children with some of these features will be accepted is low. Primary care professionals may also be left to manage children 'not unwell enough' for CAMHS.

Despite this, there are some presentations where a more immediate mental health referral should be considered (Box 26.4).

Self-harm/suicide risk

Self-harm is defined as any act of self-poisoning or self-injury carried out by an individual irrespective of motivation. It is frequently a way of coping with or expressing overwhelming emotional distress.

Self-harm is common in young people, with at least 10% reporting having self-harmed. There can also be important consequences from self-harm, and it can result in medical complications, infection, permanent scarring or organ damage (as in the case of paracetamol overdoses).

Risk factors for self-harm include the following:

- Sex: self-harm is more common in females than males, especially in early adolescence
- Sexual and gender identity: rates of mental health disorder, self-harm and suicide are much higher in the lesbian, gay, bisexual, transgender/transsexual plus (LGBT+) community.
- Coexisting mental health disorder: 11–16-year-olds with a mental health disorder were more likely to have self-harmed or attempted suicide at some point compared to those without a disorder (25.5% vs 3%)
- Coexisting NDD

The lifetime risk of completed suicide is 50–100 times greater for someone who has self-harmed previously compared with someone who has not, thus self-harm carries a significant risk of future suicidal behaviours.

Self-harm falls into two categories:

- Self-injury with intent to die – suicidal behaviours
- Self-injury without intent to die – non-suicidal self-injury (NSSI), which is deliberate destruction of one's own body tissue without suicidal intent and for purposes not socially accepted (e.g. tattooing or piercing)

Common methods of self-harm include:

- Biting
- Hitting
- Burning
- Head banging
- Pinching
- Rubbing
- Scratching
- Self-poisoning (e.g. medication overdose)
- Self-cutting

Confidentiality is an important consideration – at the earliest opportunity it is important to let the young person know what you can and cannot keep confidential. It is vital not to promise confidentiality when this is not appropriate, but even if you need to disclose some information, it should be the minimum necessary for the young person's safety.

Remember to take the young person somewhere private for this consultation and accept that it may be very difficult or distressing for them to talk.

Assessing self-harm

Assessment of self-harm should include the following:

- General medical history – consider chronic pain and chronic physical health problems
- Full history of the behaviour, including:
  - Age of onset
  - Incidence over time; specific aspects of the behaviour over time
  - History of method(s)
  - Frequency
  - Location(s)
  - Number of injuries per episode
  - Medical severity of injuries
  - Sleep, appetite, concentration and energy levels
- Associated psychiatric comorbidities, e.g. ADHD, anxiety, autism, learning difficulties/disabilities, depression, alcohol, substance misuse, eating disorders

Bear in mind that certain variables (e.g. frequency/numbers of injuries) may change with time, increasing in severity or waxing and waning to reflect periods of stress.

Be aware that children who self-harm may be trying to elicit/express certain things:

- Attempting to elicit care
- Expressing emotion (e.g. hurt)
- Trying to 'escape' or to 'feel something'

- Expressing low self-esteem
- Managing emotional upset
- Reducing tension
- Regaining control over feelings
- Expressing a sense of hopelessness
- Trying to punish themselves

Potential family factors that may be present in children who self-harm include:

- Abuse/neglect
- Alcohol/substance problems in family
- Family history of self-harm
- Parental mental health problems
- Poor family relationship/conflict, including domestic abuse

Potential social factors that may be present in children who self-harm:

- Difficult peer relationships
- Bullying (including cyberbullying)
- Use of social media
- Identification with peer group/friends who self-harm

Asking a young person about reasons for self-harming can be tricky and the use of open-ended questions can help (Box 26.5). There are also red flags to look out for when considering referral to CAMHS (Box 26.6).

It is important to distinguish between NSSI and suicidal behaviours. NSSI may be similar to and co-occur in those with other mental health issues and should be effectively assessed and monitored.

Rare/uncommon syndromes can occur with NSSI (although not all young people who self-harm will need screening):

- Lesch-Nyhan syndrome
- Fragile X syndrome
- Cornelia de Lange syndrome
- Prader-Willi syndrome
- Retts syndrome

Box 26.5 **How to Elicit Reasons Behind Self-Harming Behaviour**

- 'Can you tell me about how you came to start harming yourself?'
- If an overdose was taken, find out what was taken, how much, at what time and if there was any use of alcohol or drugs
- 'How were you feeling at the time?'
- 'How did it make you feel afterwards?'
- 'Did you tell anyone afterwards?'
- 'Do you think we need to worry about your safety?'

Box 26.6 **Red Flag Symptoms and Signs in Risk Assessment**

Ask about:
- Specific suicidal plans:
  - Has the young person written a suicide note?
  - Have they have carried out any final acts (e.g. given away prized possessions)?
  - Were there attempts at concealment/were medications stockpiled?
- Hopelessness
- Dangerous methods used:
  - Strangulation
  - Hanging
  - Use of motor vehicles
- Ongoing suicidal intent:
  - How do they feel now that the suicide attempt failed?
  - Do they have ongoing active or passive suicidal feelings?
  - Do they want to try again?
  - Do they have the means to try again?
  - Is there anything that will stop them trying again?
- Consider using the HEEADSSSS assessment tool to help shape suitable questions:
  - Home environment
  - Education and employment (e.g. any history of non-attendance)
  - Eating (e.g. if appetite has changed)
  - Activities (peer related)
  - Drugs
  - Sexuality
  - Suicide/depression
  - Safety from injury and violence
  - Sleep (e.g. changes in)

Conclusion

Eliciting a history and conducting an assessment with children takes time and practice. Using screening questionnaires and working collaboratively with parents or carers can assist in opening up tricky topics of conversation.

Further reading

National Institute for Health and Care Excellence (2019). Depression in children and young people: identification and management. NICE Guideline [NG134]. https://www.nice.org.uk/guidance/ng134

National Institute for Health and Care Excellence (2022). Self-harm: assessment, management and preventing recurrence. NICE Guideline [NG225]. https://www.nice.org.uk/guidance/ng225/chapter/Recommendations#risk-assessment-tools-and-scales

CHAPTER 27

Treating Mental Health Conditions in Children and Young People with Neurodevelopmental Disorders

Monica Shaha and Mini Pillay

> **OVERVIEW**
>
> - The treatment of psychiatric comorbidity in neurodevelopmental disorders (NDDs) is multimodal, incorporating medication, psychological and 'social' interventions.
> - Identifying and addressing a child's needs in relation to an NDD can have a preventative role in the development of psychiatric comorbidity.
> - The treatment of comorbid psychiatric conditions follows the same guidance overall as for children without NDDs, but has to be adapted based on the individual child's needs and available evidence base.
> - Addressing sleep difficulties should be part of managing mental health issues.
> - Managing self-harm requires a holistic approach, addressing acute and chronic biomedical and psychosocial issues collectively.

In general, the treatment of mental health comorbidities in children with neurodevelopmental conditions is complex (this chapter focuses mainly on those mentioned in the previous chapters). In conditions such as attention deficit hyperactivity disorder (ADHD) and tic disorders, where the core symptoms can be treated, doing so can lead to a reduction in psychiatry comorbidity. For example, the symptoms of anxiety in a child with ADHD are often reduced by optimising the treatment of ADHD. Similarly, while many mental health issues can lead to abnormal sleeping patterns, dysregulated sleep itself can have a negative impact on mental health and managing it more effectively should be part of a comprehensive approach to care.

The broad options for treatment are:
- Psychological interventions
- Medication
- Other interventions that do not fit those two categories

A number of evidence-based medications and psychological interventions are available to manage psychiatry comorbidities (Table 27.1).

Psychological interventions

The most commonly used, evidence-based types of therapy are cognitive behaviour therapy (CBT) and psychotherapy.

CBT can be used in young children. It teaches them to examine and change the way they think (cognition), act (behaviour) and feel (emotions). It is typically used in anxiety, depression, eating disorders and OCD. Behavioural activation is a commonly used technique whereby one identifies the activities one values the most, establishes goals around these activities and prioritises the ones to work on first. This list is then broken down into more easily achievable steps.

Types of psychotherapy include the following:
- Psychodynamic – focuses on early childhood experiences and relationships with others that can affect one's development. It is typically used in anxiety, depression and for physical symptoms thought to have a psychological basis.
- Play – a non-directed type of therapy that allows a child a safe and secure space in order to express their feelings through the medium of the activity.
- Family therapy – working with the family to identify strengths and goals, focusing on the importance of communication. It is typically used in eating disorders and problems with anger/oppositional behaviours.
- Dialectical behaviour therapy (DBT) – shows some effectiveness in individuals with severe non-suicidal self-injury and co-occurring suicidal behaviours. This approach is intensive and requires a therapist trained in DBT. Less intensive approaches that incorporate mindfulness, distress tolerance, emotion regulation and interpersonal skills may also be effective.
- Exposure response prevention – uses the techniques of habituation and extinction to target, reduce and eliminate compulsive behaviours in OCD.

Alongside medication and psychological treatments to support children with NDDs with associated mental health diagnoses, there are many other areas of support for a child:

ABC of Neurodevelopmental Disorders, First Edition. Edited by Munib Haroon.
© 2024 John Wiley & Sons Ltd. Published 2024 by John Wiley & Sons Ltd.

Table 27.1 Interventions in psychiatric comorbidities of neurodevelopmental disorders.

Diagnosis	Psychological intervention	Medication	Overview of treatment
Anxiety disorders	Cognitive behaviour therapy (CBT)	No medication is licensed for use for anxiety in under-18s in the United Kingdom, but multiple randomised controlled trials support the use of selective serotonin reuptake inhibitors (SSRIs) either alone or in combination with CBT. Sertraline, which is licensed for obsessive compulsive disorder (OCD) is commonly used	Stepped model of treatment Psychological interventions are first line Medication, if used, should be in combination with psychological interventions
Depressive disorders	CBT	Fluoxetine is licensed in children over the age of 8 years	Stepped model of treatment Psychological interventions are first line Medication, if used, should be in combination with psychological interventions
Eating disorders (anorexia nervosa)	Cognitive behavioural therapy for eating disorders (CBT-ED) Family therapy Psychotherapy	Getting adequate nutrition is the generally accepted treatment for anorexia nervosa If other symptoms persist on weight restoration, e.g. anxiety/depression, then these can be treated as above	No medication has been shown to be effective for the treatment of the core features of anorexia nervosa
Schizophrenia spectrum and other psychotic disorders	Family intervention with individual CBT	Marketing authorisation for antipsychotics in under-18s varies widely Treatment decisions should be made on a case-by-case basis, considering other factors such as physical health Aripiprazole, a commonly used antipsychotic, is licensed for ages 15 years and over Others include risperidone, amisulpride and planzapine Most of these are not licensed in under-18s	Confirmed cases of psychosis should be treated with antipsychotics in conjunction with psychological interventions
OCD	CBT Exposure response prevention Involving family or carers	SSRIs have shown efficacy in treating OCD Sertraline is licensed in ages 6 and above Fluvoxamine is licensed in ages 8 and above	Stepped care model of treatment is followed First line is psychological interventions Medication is used in conjunction with psychological interventions
Sleep difficulties	Sleep hygiene Meditation Progressive muscle relaxation	Melatonin (licensed and unlicensed forms are available)	Non-pharmacological strategies should be tried first in general
Conduct disorder, oppositional defiant disorder	Parent training programme Social and cognitive problem-solving programmes Multisystemic therapy	Treat any comorbidity, especially attention deficit hyperactivity disorder Risperidone (licensed from 5 years of age) for the short-term management of severely aggressive behaviour that has not responded to psychosocial interventions	Do not offer pharmacological interventions for the routine management of behavioural problems in children and young people with oppositional defiant disorder or conduct disorder

- Support from other parents – groups across the United Kingdom offer information and support to parents whose children have NDDs and are affected by childhood mental health difficulties.
- Financial support – based on a child's needs, families may be entitled to financial support, e.g. Disability Living Allowance.
- Educational input – based on a child's needs, parents can request specific support in school.
- Social care input – early help, usually coordinated by local social care agencies, offers support to families when a problem first occurs.
- Caring for carers – as important as medication and therapy. Supporting and empowering parents to look after themselves are important.
- Information – waiting times for accessing therapy are a contentious issue. There are many resources available via the internet that can be pursued while a child is awaiting formal therapy.
- Specific organisations that offer help and support to families with diagnosed conditions include Anxiety UK (www.anxietyuk.org.uk),

OCD Action (https://ocdaction.org.uk), BEAT (www.beateatingdisorders.org.uk) and Tourette's Action UK (www.tourettes-action.org.uk).

Medication

When prescribing psychotropic medication for children and adolescents, there are certain considerations to be kept in mind (Box 27.1). In addition, deciding when to use medication and when to stick to psychological interventions requires some thought (Box 27.2).

Managing sleep difficulties

Sleep difficulties should be assessed carefully, as there can be many multifactorial reasons for their presence, not all of which are biologically mediated. For example, noise, stress, habit, light (natural and artificial) and heat can all play a part, as can the

Box 27.1 **Key considerations when prescribing medication**

- Medication is only one component of treatment.
- Inform parents and give developmentally appropriate information to the child/young person about the medication, including its purpose, nature, likely effects and risks, chances of success and the availability of other options.
- Obtain informed consent from the parent and from the child/young person where appropriate. Consider whether the child/young person has capacity to consent (if over 16 years of age) or is 'Gillick competent' (if under 16).
- Inform parents and the young person if medication is being used off-label, i.e. whether the medication has/has not been approved for children and adolescents with the condition (and according to other parameters, e.g. age/weight) for which it is being prescribed.
- 'Start low, go slow' when titrating medication upwards.
- Avoid abrupt discontinuation if medication has been taken for an extended period.
- If the child's emotions/behaviours change on the medication, do not assume this is necessarily due to the medication or due to the medication alone. Enquire about other factors, including stress, changes in the environment, physical illness and specific efforts by the child/young person, family and others to improve functioning.
- Avoid using more than one medication for the same condition (i.e. polypharmacy).

Box 27.2 **Therapy versus medication: how do we choose?**

- Severity of symptoms – general advice from the National Institute for Health and Care Excellence (NICE) is that minor symptoms are more responsive to psychological interventions. More severe symptoms may respond better to a combination of medication and therapy.
- Patient choice – children and/or their parents may express their wish to start with medication before therapy. This may be acceptable in some circumstances, but in arriving at an agreement the clinician should explain the pros and cons of both, including the evidence base and what is generally accepted practice within the United Kingdom. Discussions should be documented.
- Evidence base – this is changing, but national guidance is a starting point.
- Availability of treatments – accessibility to therapy can be hindered by waiting lists.
- Not one size fits all – the most important aspect of managing a child's mental health is working collaboratively with the child and their family. Parents know their children better than anyone and it is important to take their wishes into account. There is no 'one size fits all' treatment package for children with ADHD, for example; each child with ADHD has a unique set of strengths and struggles that can respond differently to help and support. Regularly monitoring how a child is doing is essential.

presence of NDDs, mental health conditions and other medical problems (like sleep apnoea or asthma). Explanations should be sought via a careful history and examination, as required.

Part of this includes a sleep history. Factors to take into account include:

- Evidence of sleep deprivation (e.g. falling asleep in the day, difficulty with concentration, increased irritability)
- What time is bedtime? Is there an irregular sleep habit?
- Bedtime routine, e.g. bath, drink, food
- Use of gadgets – TV, phone, iPad
- Time taken to fall asleep
- Does the child wake during the night – if so, how many times and how is this managed?
- What time does the child wake to start the day?
- Enquiries about physical health and mental well-being, the control of any NDD symptoms and looking for other factors that may explain sleep difficulties
- Set-up at home, e.g. when the family go to bed, who shares bedrooms, what the surroundings are like, e.g. whether the room is too bright/hot/noisy, what has been tried to minimise this, e.g. blackout blinds
- Exercise and physical activity history
- Substances that could interfere with sleep: medication and food/drink history (e.g. use of caffeine, ADHD medication)

In general, condition-specific guidelines should be followed, such as NICE's guidance on autism. The underlying issue should always be addressed, for example an underlying medical condition or the presence of an environmental trigger, but there are simple strategies that can help with promoting sleep:

- Regular sleep/wake schedule – this can be crucial
- Right temperature – e.g. room temperature not too warm or too cold
- Bedrooms are for sleeping – not for reading, studying, watching TV
- Promote the use of sleep-inducing foods around bedtime, e.g. milk, cheese, bananas, pistachios
- Avoid caffeine in the evening
- Relaxing routine – this may include a bath, reading, music or white noise
- Sensory stimulation – this may require fewer unpleasant or distracting stimulants and more of those that help relax

In managing sleep difficulties, getting parents to keep a sleep diary for two weeks can be helpful, as can coming up with a sleep plan that can be referred to at regular intervals.

Medication for sleep difficulties in children/adolescents

Prescribing of medication to induce sleep should be in line with the British National Formulary (BNF) and be done as per national guidance (for example, in autism this is when behavioural interventions are not working and sleep problems are having a negative impact on the child/young person and their family/carers). There is a risk of habituation with prolonged use. There are a limited number of medications used to induce sleep (Table 27.2). The medication's summary of product characteristics should be consulted.

Self-harm

It can be tricky for children to open up about their struggles, perhaps more so if they have associated NDDs (see Chapter 26 and Box 26.5).

Table 27.2 Medications for sleep used in children/adolescents.

Medication	UK Licensing	Additional notes
Antihistamines – promethazine	Not licensed to treat insomnia in children Licensed for short-term use as a paediatric sedative (e.g. for procedures)	Contraindicated <2 years of age, due to potential for fatal respiratory depression Could cause drowsiness the next day Sedative effect may diminish after a few days of continued use
Melatonin	Slenyto, a prolonged-release form of melatonin, is licensed to treat insomnia in children 2–18 years old with autism and/or Smith-Magenis syndrome where behavioural measures have not worked Adaflex®, an immediate-release preparation, can be used in children and adolescents (6–17 years old) with attention deficit hyperactivity disorder, where other healthy sleeping routines have not worked well enough	Reduces time to fall asleep ('sleep latency') May cause drowsiness Long-term effects on children are not known Off-label use of medication is often seen, for example Circadin® (which is licensed for use in adults) in children with autism who have sleep difficulties
Chloral hydrate	Chloral hydrate	Not generally recommended outside its use as a sedative for procedures Needs specialist supervision

Treatment will need to be conducted in an appropriate setting and suitable local referral pathways should be consulted. The following principles should be noted:

- Young people who have self-harmed will likely be in acute distress.
- Treat wounds (e.g. cuts, burns) in the same way you would treat accidental wounds:
  ○ Give appropriate pain relief and local anaesthesia if necessary.
  ○ Ask whether the young person thinks they are likely to interfere with wound healing (this might guide the choice of sutures or glue).
  ○ Be careful of using bandages, which can be used as ligatures.
- For a suspected overdose, once a toxin has been identified consult TOXBASE (UK National Poisons Information Service, www.toxbase.org) for appropriate treatment.
- While the priority has to be physical needs (e.g. managing an overdose, major blood loss, burns or trauma), a psychosocial assessment should not be delayed until after medical treatment is complete.
- Treating children and young people with respect, compassion and dignity is essential to earn their trust.
- Allowing a safe space for disclosure, listening without judgement and taking a holistic approach to care focusing on physical (managing any acute injuries), social and psychological aspects of care is good practice.

- All self-harm in children and young people should be taken seriously.
- Clear communication and explanation of treatment can make a young person and their family feel more at ease and involved in their care.
- Where concerns arise about care quality or significant harm, joint assessment by social care and health services staff should be arranged, with local procedures to reflect this.
- Children and young people who have acutely self-harmed should be assessed by healthcare professionals experienced in the assessment of children and young people who self-harm.

Interventions for Self-harm

When planning treatment following self-harm, professionals should take into account the outcome of any psychosocial assessments carried out and the presence of coexisting conditions. Condition-specific guidance should be followed where possible. Interventions can be increasingly specialised (Box 27.3).

Safe discharge from hospital is important, and there are several things to consider before discharging a patient (Figure 27.1), including:

- Medical and psychological fitness – both medical and mental health teams need to agree that the child/young person is safe to leave.
- Place of discharge – are they going to a safe place? Are they going back to a supportive environment or one that might trigger further self-harm?
- Follow-up plans – what is being put in place to change the circumstances that led to self-harm? Are the mental health services going to remain involved and review the patient quickly?

Box 27.3 **Interventions for self-harm**

- Regular risk assessment is essential; be aware that the degree of risk may change with time
- Individual strengths-based approach – to identify solutions for reducing distress
- Behavioural activation – practising behaviours to elicit a positive emotional state
- Self-help techniques:
- Distraction (e.g. go for a walk, draw/write something, keep a diary, stroke a pet, watch a film, get in touch with a friend, listen to music)
- Releasing emotions (e.g. clench an ice cube, snap an elastic band on wrist, exercise, draw on skin with red pen, use a punchbag)
- Devise a crisis plan with the young person and parents/carers that may include examples of self-help strategies; people to contact when in distress; creating a hope box – with photos of happy memories, nice things people have said
- Dialectical behaviour therapy (DBT)
- Cognitive behaviour therapy (CBT)
- Medication may be offered if comorbid mental health disorders are evident (e.g. antidepressants) under the supervision of specialist mental health professionals, but not as a specific intervention to reduce self-harm

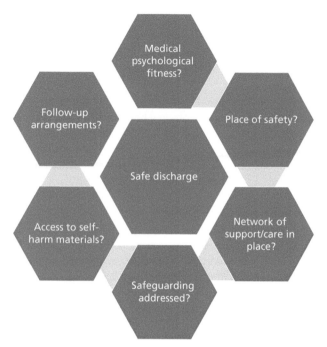

Figure 27.1 Considerations for safe discharge from hospital.

- Interdisciplinary working – its presence at the earliest opportunity is also key to supporting the young person. This should include the GP, school, Child and Adolescent Mental Health Services (CAMHS; if appropriate) and any other agencies (e.g. voluntary) that may be involved. Crucially, parents/carers must always be involved unless clear safeguarding concerns suggest that the parents/carers are the trigger.

- Support – what support does the young person have? Parents, family, friends, school or professionals? Is there someone that they feel comfortable going to if they need to talk? Do they have a way of reaching out in an emergency?
- Safeguarding – have any safeguarding concerns been addressed? If necessary, have social services been contacted?
- Access to further methods of self-harm – it is impossible to remove every single possible method of self-harm, or for a young person to be constantly supervised. However, parents should be advised to keep medications locked away to discourage impulsive overdoses.

Further reading

American Association of Child and Adolescent Psychiatry (2012). A guide for community child serving agencies on psychotropic medications for children and adolescents. https://www.aacap.org/App_Themes/AACAP/docs/press/guide_for_community_child_serving_agencies_on_psychotropic_medications_for_children_and_adolescents_2012.pdf

Effective Child Therapy (2022). Evidence-Based Therapies. https://effectivechildtherapy.org/therapies

National Institute for Health and Care Excellence (NICE) (2011). Autism spectrum disorder in under 19s: recognition, referral and diagnosis. Clinical guideline [CG128]. https://www.nice.org.uk/guidance/cg128

National Institute for Health and Care Excellence (NICE) (2014). Anxiety disorders. NICE quality standard [QS53]. https://www.nice.org.uk/guidance/qs53

National Institute for Health and Care Excellence (NICE) (2022). Self-harm: assessment, management and preventing recurrence. NICE guideline [NG225]. https://www.nice.org.uk/guidance/ng225

National Institute for Health and Care Excellence (NICE) (2023). British National Formulary for Children (BNFC). https://bnfc.nice.org.uk

CHAPTER 28

Adult Mental Health in Neurodevelopmental Disorders: Autism

Conor Davidson and Sharmi Ghosh

> **OVERVIEW**
>
> - Autistic adults are much more likely to experience mental health problems than the general population.
> - Some studies suggest a neurobiological basis for the association between autism and mental health difficulties.
> - Having to overcome life barriers and deal with mutual miscommunications and misunderstandings due to societal misconceptions may make autistic adults more prone to mental health difficulties.
> - Autistic people consistently report difficulties accessing appropriate mental health support.
> - Professionals working with autistic people should be adequately trained, and services should make reasonable adjustments to help alleviate access issues.

Autistic adults are much more likely to experience a range of mental health problems than the general population. This chapter discusses this concern, puts forward some theories for why it is so, and summarises the most common mental health disorders that co-occur with autism, with an emphasis on how presentation and treatment may differ from a neurotypical patient. Finally, tips on making reasonable adjustments for autistic patients in mental health settings are described.

Incidence of mental health disorders in adult autism

The research evidence in this area tends to be of poor methodological quality, being mainly based on specialist clinic convenience samples. Different studies give widely divergent estimates of rates of co-occurring conditions: for example, the co-occurrence of schizophrenia with adult autism ranges from 0% to 30%, depending on the study. In recent years, systematic reviews and meta-analyses have brought more clarity. In our view, a conservative assumption is that at least one-third of adults with autism will have another diagnosable psychiatric condition. Multiple comorbidity is also more common compared to the general population, with many autistic people having two or more co-occurring psychiatric conditions.

Exactly why autistic people are more prone to mental health problems is not entirely clear. Some studies have shown certain genetic and neuroanatomical variations in the neurodivergent population, perhaps indicating a similar neurobiological basis for autism and some mental health disorders.

In our view, however, most of the increased incidence of mental health issues in the autistic population can be ascribed to two factors:

- Due to their unique way of perceiving the world around them (Figure 28.1), individuals with autism have to overcome more life barriers than neurotypicals. This can lead to fatigue, disillusionment and demotivation. The result can be diminished quality of relationships and friendships, and academic and professional underachievement. All of these are already known to be risk factors for poor mental health.
- Society at large is still learning to accommodate the uniqueness of the neurodivergent. Mutual miscommunications and misunderstandings can lead to breakdown of support, negative feedback and even ostracism for perceived deviation from societal norms. These factors, if not addressed through effective adjustments, accommodations and understanding from others, again cause deterioration in mental health.

Regardless of the cause, it is certain that all mental health practitioners will see many autistic patients in the course of their clinical practice. Again, the research evidence here is of mixed quality; however, it is reasonable to assume that 1 in 25 psychiatric outpatients and 1 in 10 inpatients with be autistic. Despite this, autistic people frequently report difficulty accessing mental health services and poor experiences of mental health treatment. Outcomes tend to be worse as well; for example, rates of completed suicide in autism are at least seven times higher than in the general population. From clinical experience we postulate three reasons for this situation:

- Because of issues with communication and social interaction, people with autism might be disadvantaged in seeking the help that they need.

ABC of Neurodevelopmental Disorders, First Edition. Edited by Munib Haroon.
© 2024 John Wiley & Sons Ltd. Published 2024 by John Wiley & Sons Ltd.

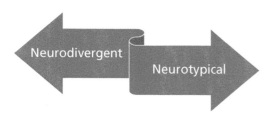

Figure 28.1 Neurodivergent and neurotypical people can perceive the world around them differently. For those in the minority – the neurodivergent – this can lead to more barriers and create the potential for mutual miscommunication and misunderstanding.

Box 28.1 **The most common mental health issues seen in autism**

- Depressive disorders
- Anxiety disorders
- Obsessive compulsive and related disorders
- Bipolar and related disorders
- Schizophrenia spectrum/psychotic disorders
- Substance-related and addictive disorders
- Feeding and eating disorders
- Personality disorders

- Presentation of mental health issues can be slightly different in individuals with autism and there is a risk of subtle signs being missed on a mental state examination.
- Most mental health practitioners, at least in the United Kingdom, tend to have relatively poor understanding and limited clinical experience of adult autism.

An interesting point to note here is that in order to deal with the stress of the everyday world, some people with autism employ a technique known as camouflaging. It involves learned strategies used to attenuate or 'mask' non-normative differences in their behaviour. A common example is 'training' oneself to make eye contact every few seconds during conversation. A systematic review of this phenomenon has shown that when the rate of self-reported camouflaging is higher, the mental health outcomes are worse.

The common mental health issues seen in autism are shown in Box 28.1 and detailed next.

Depressive disorders

At least one-third of autistic adults experience clinically significant low mood in their lifetime. Compared to the neurotypical population, autistic people tend to have fewer friends and other social contacts, are more likely to be unemployed/have financial problems and are at greater risk of traumatic events such as bullying, physical assault and sexual abuse. All of these are risk factors for depression.

Autistic people often have difficulty describing emotions and feelings. They may struggle to understand an open/ambiguous question like 'How are you feeling today?' Therefore, clinicians should be alert to objective signs of depression such as weight loss

and psychomotor retardation (slow movements). One possible presenting feature of depression that seems unique to autism is an increase in stereotyped and repetitive behaviour, typically accompanied by decreased social activity.

Treatment of depressive illness in autistic people should proceed along existing best practice clinical guidelines, ideally with both cognitive behavioural therapy (CBT) and a selective serotonin reuptake inhibitor (SSRI) antidepressant used in conjunction. Traditionally, specialist autism clinicians have tended to favour citalopram and sertraline over other antidepressants, but there is little firm research evidence to back up this clinical intuition (the first large-scale multicentre randomised controlled trial in adult autism is looking at sertraline versus placebo, and should report findings by 2024). It is wise to start with a lower dose of SSRI than normal, as people with autism are more prone to idiosyncratic side effects such as psychomotor over-activation.

Anxiety disorders

Along with depression, anxiety is the most common comorbid mental health issue seen in autistic adults. One large population-based study in 2020 found that anxiety disorders were diagnosed in 20.1% of adults with autism compared with 8.7% of controls, with the greatest risk for people with autism without intellectual disability.

The common difficulties with social interaction and communication seen in autism can make even everyday social situations anxiety provoking. Resistance to and difficulties in adjusting to change can also give rise to raised anxiety levels, as can 'sensory overload' in loud, busy environments. It is not uncommon in an adult neurodevelopmental clinic to find autism in individuals who have had a prior diagnosis of social anxiety/social phobia.

Note that in some autistic individuals, anxiety can present in dramatic fashion, with extreme 'meltdowns' sometimes involving aggression to property, themselves or others.

Treatment of anxiety disorders in adult autism is similar to the recommendations earlier for treating depression, although CBT tends to be considered first line before SSRI medication. It is important that the CBT therapist has an understanding of autism and is able to adapt their communication style and treatment strategies accordingly. In psychotherapy settings, autistic clients tend to respond best to clear communication, explicit treatment goals and an emphasis on practical behavioural change (as opposed to reframing cognitions).

Obsessive compulsive and related disorders

Obsessive compulsive disorder (OCD) in autism can present an interesting diagnostic dilemma. While OCD is more prevalent in autistic individuals compared to the general population, some features of autism overlap with those of OCD and it is possible for the inexperienced clinician to mistake one for the other. Features seen in both conditions include repetitive behaviour, rituals, fixation on routine and perfectionism.

Despite these superficially similar features, the subjective experience of autism versus OCD is very different. In autism, repetitive behaviours, intense interests and rituals provide familiarity and comfort. The individual regards them as 'the right way to do things' and has no desire to change. In psychiatry, such thoughts and behaviours are described as 'egosytonic'. In OCD, obsessive thinking and compulsive behaviours are 'egodystonic'. This means that the individual does not *want* to carry them out, but they feel they have to in order to avoid some imagined catastrophic outcome. Rather than being soothing, OCD obsessions and compulsions tend to be distressing and a source of great anxiety to the patient.

It follows that the clinical approach to autism and OCD is very different. OCD sufferers typically seek psychiatric help and are keen to change their repetitive behaviours. On the other hand, it is almost always undesirable – and sometimes downright harmful – to attempt to 'treat' autistic repetitive behaviour.

Bipolar and related disorders

Although once again the research literature must be treated with caution, it is very likely that bipolar and related disorders (BARD) are more common in autism, perhaps by as much as a factor of five. Compared to neurotypicals, autistic people with BARD seem to experience more mixed affective features (depression and mania) and fewer episodes of euphoric mood. Possible presenting features include mood lability, restlessness, irritability/aggression and psychotic symptoms. Mental state examination of an individual with autism and suspected BARD can be more challenging: for example, some autistic people habitually speak loudly and fast, which can be mistaken for the 'pressure of speech' seen in mania. As with all the psychiatric conditions described in this chapter, the examining clinician should ideally have a good understanding of the patient's 'baseline' presentation in order to detect any deviation due to mental illness.

Treatment of bipolar disorders in autistic people is a very underresearched field. Lithium therapy seems to be relatively safe and effective, although rates of gastrointestinal side effects may be higher. There is a suggestion that autistic people are more at risk of antidepressant-induced mania, although this claim requires further investigation.

Schizophrenia spectrum and other psychotic disorders

Once again, rates of psychosis and schizophrenia (a major mental illness characterised by repeated episodes of psychosis) are higher in autism. Autistic people seem to be particularly at risk of what are termed 'reactive' brief psychotic episodes during periods of great stress (often transitional times such as living away from home for the first time). Typically, such episodes will settle with time and relatively conservative treatment.

Diagnosis of schizophrenia can be complicated by the features it can share with autism: for example, social withdrawal, perceptual distortions and intensely held beliefs. Crucial differentiating factors are the presence of frank hallucinations and delusions, age of onset (it is extremely rare for symptoms of schizophrenia to present before late adolescence) and response to antipsychotic medication.

Psychiatrists should be cautious in their treatment approach. Autistic people are more prone to side effects from antipsychotic drugs. There have been cases of serious motor side effects, neuroleptic malignant syndrome and even death. The axiom 'start low and go slow' (in terms of medication dose) particularly applies here.

Substance-related and addictive disorders

Early research suggested that autistic people were less likely to develop problematic drug and alcohol use, perhaps because of diminished peer influence and greater tendency to ruleboundedness. However, more recent evidence shows that in fact rates of alcohol misuse – and probably illicit drug misuse as well – are higher in the population of those with autism.

Common reasons for substance misuse include to help cope with life stressors, family history of addiction and comorbid mental health issues. All of these hold true for autistic individuals. Furthermore, the day-to-day social struggles of an autistic person can lead to their seeking relief with drugs or alcohol. It is not unusual in our clinic for autistic people to report that they routinely drink alcohol to cope with quotidian social interactions. Because autistic people are drawn to routine and repetition, alcohol (or drug) use can quickly become stereotyped and excessive.

On the more positive side, there is some evidence to suggest that autistic people with alcohol dependence are better able to achieve total abstinence than neurotypicals, perhaps because *do not drink alcohol at all under any circumstances* is a very clear, 'black-and-white' rule to follow. One treatment consideration to bear in mind is that some autistic people may not be well suited to '12-step' peer support programmes such as Alcoholics Anonymous, as such groups typically require a high degree of social interaction.

Feeding and eating disorders

In recent years there has been growing interest in the high rates of eating disorders seen in autism. Interestingly, often the presenting features are more akin to avoidant restrictive food intake disorder (ARFID) rather than classical anorexia nervosa. These might include preference for or avoidance of a particular food/food groups depending on sensory qualities like texture, smell or colour. A strong preference for routine and familiarity can mean that meal times and recipes are very fixed. Often autistic people find it difficult to eat food unless it is arranged in a specific order on their plate, or they prefer a specific plate or spoon to eat with. The social aspect of eating food together is not a comfortable experience for some; others may struggle with physical difficulties like problems with eating and chewing.

The treatment of eating disorders in autistic people may require significant adaptations to account for the issues described here. It can be a clinical challenge sometimes to differentiate autistic features from eating disorder symptoms: for example, distinguishing sensory issues precluding certain food textures from the more generalised avoidance of food seen in anorexia nervosa. The Pathway for Eating disorders and Autism developed from Clinical Experience (PEACE) resources (www.peacepathway.org) are a useful reference point for clinicians working in this area.

Personality disorders

The interface between personality disorder and autism is one of the most interesting and controversial in modern psychiatry. In recent years there has been growing concern about the widespread misdiagnosis of autistic people (particularly young females) with borderline personality disorder (also known as emotionally unstable personality disorder). The research evidence for this claim is perhaps lagging behind expert clinical opinion, but without doubt we have seen a number of such examples in our own practice. Unfortunately the debate can become polarised at times, losing sight of the fact that real-life psychiatric diagnosis is always a little 'blurry round the edges'.

We anticipate that the revised classification system for personality disorder in ICD-11 (which came into effect in 2022) will add to the confusion in this area. Two of the key criteria for diagnosing personality disorder in ICD-11 are problems with the 'ability to develop and maintain close and mutually satisfying relationships' and with the 'ability to understand others' perspectives', both of which are commonly seen in autism. Furthermore, the newly revised 'prominent personality disorder traits or patterns' section includes 'detachment' and 'anankastia' subtypes, both of which show considerable overlap with core features of autism.

In daily practice, it can be a challenge to distinguish between autism and personality disorder. Markers of personality disorder may include severe and prolonged childhood trauma; severe and persistent self-harming behaviour; antisocial behaviour; and a strong counter-transference reaction (i.e. the patient displays high levels of emotional arousal that are then experienced in attenuated form by the clinician). Diagnosticians should be mindful that it is not a binary situation, and some patients have both autism and co-occurring personality disorder. The Coventry Grid can be a useful tool to guide diagnostic decision making in such cases.

Development of bespoke treatments for co-occurring autism and personality disorder is very much in its infancy, although there are some promising preliminary results for radically open dialectical behavioural therapy.

Reasonable adjustments in mental health settings

The leading autism researcher William Mandy wrote in 2022: 'The autism mental health crisis can be described with the following paradox: autistic people have a high chance of developing mental health problems but a low chance of receiving effective help.' Autistic people consistently report difficulties accessing appropriate mental health support. It is vital that all mental health practitioners ensure they are adequately trained in autism and able to make adaptations to their practice for autistic patients.

'Reasonable adjustments' is a term used in the UK Equality Act 2010. They are changes that health and social care providers are legally obliged to make to ensure that people with disabilities (including neurodevelopmental conditions like autism) are not disadvantaged compared to people without disabilities. In practice, reasonable adjustments should be personalised to the individual rather than generically applied. That said, we have provided a (non-exhaustive) list of the most common reasonable adjustments in mental health settings in Table 28.1. A good starting point is to ask the patient 'How can I best communicate with you today?'

Table 28.1 Common reasonable adjustments in healthcare settings.

Communication	Clinical	Environmental
Clear, unambiguous language	Make explicit treatment goals	Minimise ambient noise
Information given in writing as well as verbally	Give advance notice of any changes to treatment plan or personnel	Dimmable lighting
Explain clearly what will happen in the clinic appointment	Practice caution with psychotropic prescribing: *start low and go slow*	Provide sensory objects/fidget toys

Further reading

Cook, J., Hull, L., Crane, L., and Mandy, W. (2021). Camouflaging in autism: a systematic review. *Clinical Psychology Review* 89: 102080.

Cox, C., Bulluss, E., Chapman, F. et al. (2019). The Coventry Grid for adults: a tool to guide clinicians in differentiating complex trauma and autism. *Good Autism Practice* 20 (1): 76–87.

Hollocks, M.J., Lerh, J.W., Magiati, I. et al. (2019). Anxiety and depression in adults with autism spectrum disorder: a systematic review and meta-analysis. *Psychological Medicine* 49 (4): 559–572.

Lai, M.-C., Kassee, C., Besney, R. et al. (2019). Prevalence of co-occurring mental health diagnoses in the autism population: a systematic review and meta-analysis. *Lancet Psychiatry* 6 (10): 819–829.

Mandy, W. (2022). Six ideas about how to address the autism mental health crisis. *Autism* 26 (2): 289–292.

Nimmo-Smith, V., Heuvelman, H., Dalman, C. et al. (2020). Anxiety disorders in adults with autism spectrum disorder: a population-based study. *Journal of Autism and Developmental Disorders* 50 (1): 308–318.

Tromans, S., Chester, V., Kiani, R. et al. (2018). The prevalence of autism spectrum disorders in adult psychiatric inpatients: a systematic review. *Clinical Practice and Epidemiology in Mental Health* 14: 177–187.

CHAPTER 29

Adult Mental Health in Neurodevelopmental Disorders: Intellectual Developmental Disorder, Attention Deficit Hyperactivity Disorder, Tourette's Disorder and Other Conditions

Alwyn Kam

> **OVERVIEW**
>
> - Common mental health problems in intellectual developmental disorder (IDD) include depression, anxiety disorders and schizophrenia.
> - Recognition of IDD can be challenging due to communication and cognitive difficulties.
> - A person-centred approach to IDD is crucial, including tailored assessments and treatments.
> - Dementia occurs earlier in people with IDD, especially those with Down's syndrome.
> - Specialised assessment, management and support of IDD are often needed.
> - Attention deficit hyperactivity disorder (ADHD) is associated with higher rates of anxiety disorders, mood disorders, substance-related disorders and personality disorders.
> - Careful distinction between ADHD symptoms and mental health problems is necessary for appropriate treatment.
> - Anxiety disorders, depression and obsessive compulsive disorder are known associations of Tourette's disorder in adults.
> - There is increasing recognition that adults with conditions such as developmental coordination disorder and specific learning disorder have higher rates of mental health difficulties.
> - Proper recognition and treatment of mental health problems can improve daily functioning and overall well-being in individuals with neurodevelopmental disorders.

Mental health needs in people with neurodevelopmental disorders (NDDs) are easily overlooked. Adults with conditions such as intellectual developmental disorder (IDD), attention deficit hyperactivity disorder (ADHD), Tourette's disorder and chronic tic disorders, developmental coordination disorder and specific learning disorder may be affected by mental health disorders including depressive disorder (depression), anxiety disorders, schizophrenia spectrum and other psychotic disorders (schizophrenia and psychosis), bipolar and related disorders (bipolar disorder), dementias, feeding and eating disorders and substance-related disorders (including alcohol).

Confusion can arise, however, as some sources will classify neurodevelopmental conditions such as autism and ADHD as mental health disorders, which complicates the analysis of the prevalence of mental conditions in neurodevelopmental conditions.

The probability that someone with an NDD will experience mental health needs is dependent on the interplay of innate/biological factors (such as genetics) and extrinsic factors such as being exposed to negative life events, having limited access to resources and opportunities to learn coping skills, as well as the effect of other people's attitudes.

In broad terms, the treatment and management of mental health problems are usually the same for those with a NDD as they are for anyone else and depend on the nature and severity of the problem, and the individual's personal circumstances and preferences. These options may include cognitive behavioural therapy (CBT), psychodynamic therapy, family therapy and medications. Interventions need to be individually tailored to the person's abilities and needs.

Intellectual developmental disorder/ intellectual disability

Incidence and prevalence

Intellectual developmental disorder is commonly used interchangeably with the term 'learning disability' in the United Kingdom (this chapter will use IDD). The prevalence of IDD can vary between 1% and 3% globally. In England 2.1% of people are thought to have IDD.

There is a wide difference in prevalence rates reported for mental health problems in people with IDD because of differing methodologies in research. In population-based studies, the prevalence of mental health problems is reported to be between 14.5% and 43.8%.

ABC of Neurodevelopmental Disorders, First Edition. Edited by Munib Haroon.
© 2024 John Wiley & Sons Ltd. Published 2024 by John Wiley & Sons Ltd.

Box 29.1 **Mental health problems more common in adults with IDD**

- Depression
- Anxiety disorder
- Schizophrenia
- Bipolar disorder
- Dementia

Box 29.2 **Examples of easy-read leaflet resources available online**

Royal College of Psychiatrists learning disabilities leaflets
https://www.rcpsych.ac.uk/mental-health/problems-disorders/learning-disabilities
Easy Health mental health resources
https://www.easyhealth.org.uk/resources/category/21-mental-health
NHS South of England, A Picture of Health
http://www.apictureofhealth.southwest.nhs.uk/mental-health

In the largest prevalence study in the United Kingdom, 28.3% of adults with IDD had current mental health problems. If challenging behaviours are included in these analyses, then this figure rises to 40.9%.

Compared to people without IDD, research suggests that certain mental health problems are significantly more common (see Box 29.1), although the prevalence of each can depend on the aetiology of the IDD. However, the most common mental health problems seen in adults with IDD are depression, anxiety disorders and schizophrenia.

Recognition of a mental health concern is not always straightforward. Affected individuals may present with challenging behaviours, such as verbal/physical aggression to people or property, or self-injurious behaviours. Challenging behaviour is itself not a diagnosis and is usually the result of other underlying issues that include mental health problems. This can raise barriers in those carrying out an assessment. And when the person being assessed cannot communicate with others about why they are feeling the way they do, it becomes especially difficult to identify what the problem is and then to address finding some sort of resolution. This failure of health professionals to recognise an additional/new health problem in a person with IDD and simply to attribute it to the known condition of IDD (diagnostic overshadowing) is an important, persistent and common issue.

Assessment and treatment considerations for mental health problems

A person-centred approach should be used for anyone with an IDD and a mental health problem. A thorough assessment of needs, including biological, psychological, environmental and social factors, should be completed to tailor investigations or interventions (see Figure 29.1).

With regard to treatment, counselling and psychotherapy are under-used for people with IDD and should be considered where appropriate. Wider aspects to take into account include addressing needs and aspects around optimising communication, addressing employment (finding it, keeping it and making reasonable adjustments), social security requirements and other social factors. Optimising physical health, getting enough sleep, exercise and good food should also not be forgotten.

Due to biological differences often linked to the aetiology of a person's IDD, it is common to be more sensitive to medication side-effects. 'Start low and go slow' is the mantra to follow here and medication should be started at the lowest dose (such as for those used in children or the elderly), with a gradual titration of the dose based on clinical effectiveness.

Communication and accessible information are important components of working with people with IDD and their carers. In mental health, there are good examples of easy-read leaflets and guides that help to explain what mental health conditions are and the treatments available (see Box 29.2).

Depression and anxiety disorders in intellectual developmental disorder

While around 6% of the mainstream population experiences depression in any year, studies suggest that this affects up to 20% of people with IDD. The biopsychosocial aspects of depressive illness are important and, given differences in cognition and communication, it may be difficult for people to express their mood, thoughts or outlook about themselves or of the future. In some cases, asking the person and others who know them well about feeling sad, tearfulness and biological symptoms such as sleep and appetite can be helpful in determining the presence of a mood problem.

Anxiety can manifest in different ways and can drive a challenging behaviour presentation. It is also not easy for an anxious person to recognise that they are anxious. So for this and other reasons, taking a careful history is important. Evidence-based practice is recommended for the person-centred treatment of depression and anxiety, making reasonable adjustments as necessary.

Schizophrenia

It is recognised that rates of schizophrenia are three times higher in adults with IDD than in the general population. However, it may not always be easy to identify psychosis, and assessing a person's internal perceptual experiences can be quite challenging, particularly if there are communication or cognitive difficulties. It is often important to combine objective observations with information from people who know the person well to determine whether a behaviour represents hallucinations, delusions or paranoia (see Box 29.3). These are best understood in the context of the person's personal history, physical health and environment. If schizophrenia or psychosis is suspected, advice from mental health services or specialised intellectual disability services is recommended.

Schizophrenia itself can cause cognitive and executive function difficulties. People with IDD and comorbid schizophrenia may present with complex management problems not seen in people with schizophrenia alone. Research suggests that should patients with

PERSON-CENTRED APPROACH FOR INDIVIDUALS WITH INTELLECTUAL DISABILITY AND MENTAL HEALTH PROBLEMS

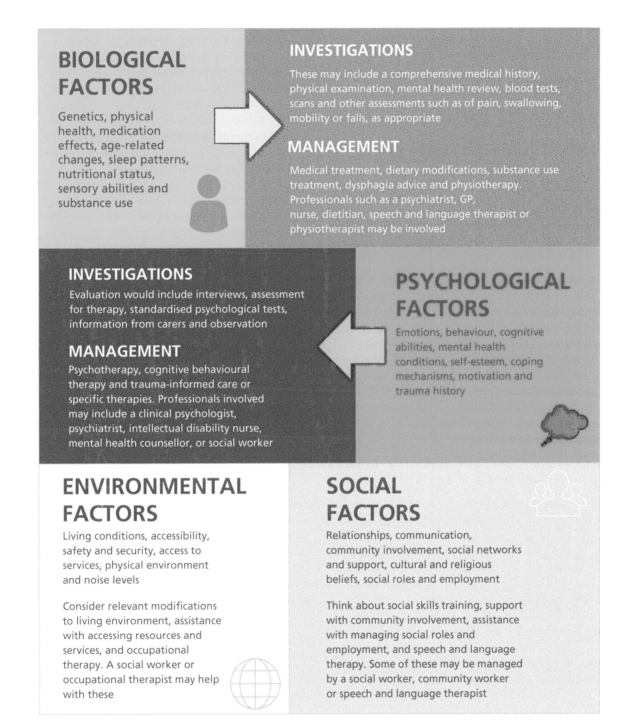

BIOLOGICAL FACTORS

Genetics, physical health, medication effects, age-related changes, sleep patterns, nutritional status, sensory abilities and substance use

INVESTIGATIONS

These may include a comprehensive medical history, physical examination, mental health review, blood tests, scans and other assessments such as of pain, swallowing, mobility or falls, as appropriate

MANAGEMENT

Medical treatment, dietary modifications, substance use treatment, dysphagia advice and physiotherapy. Professionals such as a psychiatrist, GP, nurse, dietitian, speech and language therapist or physiotherapist may be involved

INVESTIGATIONS

Evaluation would include interviews, assessment for therapy, standardised psychological tests, information from carers and observation

MANAGEMENT

Psychotherapy, cognitive behavioural therapy and trauma-informed care or specific therapies. Professionals involved may include a clinical psychologist, psychiatrist, intellectual disability nurse, mental health counsellor, or social worker

PSYCHOLOGICAL FACTORS

Emotions, behaviour, cognitive abilities, mental health conditions, self-esteem, coping mechanisms, motivation and trauma history

ENVIRONMENTAL FACTORS

Living conditions, accessibility, safety and security, access to services, physical environment and noise levels

Consider relevant modifications to living environment, assistance with accessing resources and services, and occupational therapy. A social worker or occupational therapist may help with these

SOCIAL FACTORS

Relationships, communication, community involvement, social networks and support, cultural and religious beliefs, social roles and employment

Think about social skills training, support with community involvement, assistance with managing social roles and employment, and speech and language therapy. Some of these may be managed by a social worker, community worker or speech and language therapist

Figure 29.1 An approach to assessing mental health in intellectual developmental disorder/intellectual disability.

comorbidity need psychiatric admission, the number of admissions may be lower, but their duration tends to be longer compared to individuals with schizophrenia alone. Such people are also more likely to have epilepsy, negative symptoms of schizophrenia and impairment of episodic memory, all of which have implications for antipsychotic medication dosage, adherence to treatment and efficacy.

Box 29.3 **Positive and negative symptoms of schizophrenia**

Positive symptoms	Delusions	Believing things that are not true (including persecutory thinking and paranoia)
	Hallucinations	Seeing or hearing things that are not there
	Disorganised thinking	Having thoughts that are jumbled or do not make sense
	Abnormal motor behaviour	Acting in strange or unusual ways, including catatonia
Negative symptoms	Flat affect/diminished emotional expression	Not showing emotions or feelings
	Anhedonia	Not finding joy in things that used to be enjoyed
	Avolition	Having no energy or motivation to do things (work, social or personal)
	Alogia	Speaking very little or not at all
	Asociality	Lack of interest in social interactions

Dementia (major neurocognitive disorder)

Dementias occur earlier in life in people with IDD in general. In particular, Alzheimer's disease occurs even earlier in people with Down's syndrome, due to genetic factors on Chromosome 21, with 1 in 2 people expected to be affected over the age of 60 (compared to 1 in 14 people in the general population at the same age). Recognising dementia is important, and in cases of mild IDD, symptoms may mirror those seen in the wider population. However, in more severe IDD the signs of dementia can be more elusive and might only be a non-specific change in behaviour. Differences in physical capabilities, cognitive functions or personality traits might be observed by others, and are potential triggers for a dementia assessment.

Typical dementia screening scales are often unsuitable and more specialised tools such as the Dementia Screening Questionnaire for Individuals with Intellectual Disabilities (DSQIID) can be used instead. If dementia is suspected then, as with anyone, clinical depression and reversible causes of memory problems should be rules out. This would include blood tests for vitamin B_{12} and folate deficiency, thyroid disorders, electrolytes, liver function tests, calcium, HbA1c, full blood count and erythrocyte sedimentation rate; eyesight and hearing should also be checked. Brain imaging is typically not useful unless there is a previous scan to compare it with. When dementia is suspected, a thorough assessment is recommended to establish baseline functioning, cognition and memory, either through specialised intellectual disability services or a memory service.

Attention deficit hyperactivity disorder

Incidence and prevalence

There are several mental health sequelae for adults diagnosed with ADHD as children, including increased lifetime rates of antisocial, mood, anxiety and substance-related disorders. There is a higher rate of anxiety disorders (20% compared to an 8% background risk), with impairments in psychosocial, educational and neuropsychological functioning being directly attributed to ADHD rather than their comorbidities.

ADHD is an early developmental risk factor for other mental health problems such as anxiety and depression, personality disorders (antisocial and borderline types) and substance-related disorders. Its link to schizophrenia is less defined, but it is not a strong predictor for later-life bipolar disorder. Approximately 75% of those with ADHD have another chronic health issue, with co-occurrence rates of 25–50% for depression, 60% for major depressive disorder with seasonal pattern (also known as seasonal affective disorder), 20–45% for substance-related disorders, 6–25% for personality disorders and 9% for eating disorders.

If we look at those accessing adult mental health services in the United Kingdom, we find higher rates of ADHD compared to the general population, for instance those being treated for anxiety are more than twice as likely to have ADHD as the general population. In settings such as prisons, the prevalence of ADHD has been found to be about 10 times higher than the general population prevalence. Similarly, in addiction services the occurrence of ADHD is approximately five times higher.

When assessing symptoms of mental health problems in ADHD, an initial consideration is whether the symptoms are attributable to ADHD itself, a comorbidity due to other neurodevelopmental conditions or a definite mental health condition. For example, ADHD symptoms of restlessness, avoidance behaviour, irritability, poor sleep, low self-esteem, anger, mood instability and impulsivity can mimic mental health problems and be mistaken for them.

Anxiety disorders

Anxiety can occur in many ways in an individual with ADHD. This may occur as a separate anxiety disorder, but we need also to consider that it may be directly linked to ADHD symptoms, or be an effect of ADHD medications or their withdrawal. Treatment options for individuals with both ADHD and anxiety may involve a combination of medications and psychological interventions. When considering pharmacological treatment, targeting the condition with the most severe symptoms first is usually best. However, success with psychological therapy will be higher if the core ADHD symptoms are managed first.

Mood disorders

Mood disorders can have significant impacts on a person's emotional state, whether or not they also have ADHD. These include depression presenting predominantly as low mood, bipolar disorder generally marked by extreme mood swings, and cyclothymic disorder with less severe mood changes. In seasonal affective disorder depressive episodes occur typically during the darker winter months.

Chronic low self-esteem is commonly seen as part of ADHD and typically responds to a control of symptoms and improvement in function – psychological interventions are usually helpful for this. True depressive episodes are not routinely seen as part of ADHD and would normally suggest a comorbid mental health problem. They can usually be identified by a clear change in how someone usually presents, and if present require treatment.

Mood instability in ADHD is characterised by rapid, frequent mood changes, often in response to environmental factors, manifesting as sudden irritability, frustration or excitement. This differs from affective mood disorders where mood disturbances are usually more persistent and less reactive to immediate surroundings. The mood instability seen as part of the ADHD presentation often responds to ADHD stimulant medication. It may also be mistaken for emotionally unstable personality disorder (EuPD) or bipolar disorder.

Although there are some similarities between ADHD and bipolar disorder, the former is a trait-like condition (similar to being tall or having blue eyes) and is a part of how a person is all the time, whereas bipolar disorder comes and goes with episodes of clear change followed by times when the person returns to their normal state. People with ADHD may complain of not being able to focus or sleep, whereas those with bipolar disorder can have a subjective sense of sharpened mental abilities and, in mania, a reduced need for sleep. Mood swings in ADHD are usually high frequency and low severity, lasting a shorter period of time, whereas this is less likely to be the case with bipolar disorder.

Psychosis and schizophrenia

Cognitive deficits in schizophrenia can manifest in areas such as executive function, verbal memory and attention, which are also seen in ADHD. Both conditions can present with attentional difficulties, emotional dysregulation and disorganised behaviour. Care needs be taken about confusing tangential and ceaseless, unfocused thought processes in ADHD with thought disorder, and impaired motivation and fatigue with negative symptoms in schizophrenia. However, ADHD features do not generally resemble true psychotic symptoms and insight is usually preserved in ADHD.

Schizophrenia's impact on cognitive and executive functions can intensify the difficulties experienced by a person with coexisting ADHD. Comorbidity of the two conditions can affect symptom presentation, risk and treatment. Although management is based on limited available evidence, one consideration is that prescribers of medications should be careful about the impact of any stimulant medication, particularly in those who are at high risk of developing psychosis.

Substance-related disorders

Certain genetic factors can predispose individuals to ADHD and substance use disorders, with environmental factors such as neglect and child abuse further heightening these risks. The increased probability of substance misuse may be driven in part by the presence of symptoms of impulsivity and the need to reward/stimulate dopaminergic pathways, the tendency to self-medicate and the presence of and response to negative life experiences. ADHD may also predispose to conduct disorder in childhood and antisocial personality disorder, both of which may increase the risk of substance misuse disorder.

Prescribing for people with ADHD with comorbid substance use can present a challenge. The choice of whether to medicate and what to use will depend on the type, duration and pattern of substance misuse, the presence of dependence and the possible interactions of medications with the substance. The risk of criminal offending needs to be taken into account and whether individuals want to engage with services to address their use of substances. As higher stimulant doses are needed in those with active stimulant abuse (for example, in the prison population) it is usually best to avoid using stimulant medications altogether, particularly as this may also increase the risk of psychosis. Individuals such as these need to be engaged with substance misuse services and advice for specific prescribing choices are best done in conjunction with an ADHD specialist.

Personality disorder

People with ADHD may be misdiagnosed as having a borderline personality disorder (also called EuPD) because both conditions feature difficulties with maintaining emotions, sensation seeking and impulsivity, and people with both may have unstable relationships and comorbid substance misuse. However, people with ADHD have difficulty with hyperactivity/impulsivity and inattention, whereas borderline personality disorder tends to present with abandonment avoidant behaviour and identity disturbance, with chronic feelings of emptiness and transient stress-related persecutory thoughts. Where individuals have co-occurring ADHD and personality disorder, focusing on ADHD treatment as the initial strategy can lead to improvements in inattention, impulsivity and mood swing symptoms, and the person can then benefit by engaging with psychological talking therapies to address the personality disorder.

Tourette's disorder

Tourette's disorder and chronic tic disorders are associated with a higher incidence of depression, OCD and anxiety disorders compared to the background population risk. The aetiology of these conditions is likely to be multifactorial and will vary according to phenotype, but while there will be biological factors underpinning the association, it is undoubtedly the case that people with Tourette's disorder face misunderstanding, stigma and discrimination on a frequent basis and these issues will often be contributory factors. A large proportion of people with Tourette's also have ADHD, which can complicate the clinical picture. Having Tourette's and associated mental health difficulties (as well as ADHD) can create a downward spiral of events, affecting a person's quality of life and having a detrimental impact on their familial, social and professional spheres. An increased risk of suicide in individuals with Tourette's disorder and chronic tic disorders, as well as an increased risk of death due to substance use, is described in the literature, as are an association with other physical health issues and an increased overall risk of early mortality.

Other neurodevelopmental disorders

There is ongoing research around the associations between other NDDs and mental health in children and their carers, but there is a relatively poorer evidence base in adults. It has always seemed plausible that the higher rate of mental health problems seen in children and young people could lead to continued issues as they grow older and emerging evidence appears to confirm that this is the case. For conditions like specific learning disorder and developmental coordination disorder, mental health issues could arise through a combination of a direct biological association between the condition and a mental health disorder, because of an association with another neurodevelopmental condition (such as ADHD) or because of an experiential effect, such as poor life outcomes leading to low self-esteem.

Conclusion

There is good evidence that mental health problems occur more frequently in adults with conditions like IDD, ADHD, Tourette's and autism than in people without these conditions. There is emerging evidence that this is also the case with other NDDs. Mental health problems need to be recognised before they can be managed and treated. However, they can often go unrecognised if the severity of difficulties is perceived as less than it actually is. Particularly in people with IDD, symptoms and consequential challenging behaviour may be attributed to their IDD instead of another health condition. Diagnostic overshadowing can result in unnecessarily prolonging the distress for the individual.

Increasing levels of impairment are associated with greater physical and mental health problems; this correlation is strongest in those with the most significant disabilities. The presence of co-occurring NDDs compounds comorbidity.

Proper identification and treatment of mental health concerns in individuals with neurodevelopmental conditions can lead to improved daily functioning, better outcomes in education and occupation, and improved chances of forming and maintaining relationships. They can also reduce the burden on caregivers and families. It is therefore important for healthcare professionals and caregivers to be aware of the signs of mental health problems. Research in this area needs to be continued in order to improve our understanding of the intersection of neurodevelopmental conditions and mental health.

Further reading

Alexander-Passe, N. (2015). *Dyslexia and Mental Health*. London: Jessica Kingsley Publishers.

Asherson, P. (2005). Clinical assessment and treatment of attention deficit hyperactivity disorder in adults. *Expert Review of Neurotherapeutics* 5 (4): 525–539. https://doi.org/10.1586/14737175.5.4.525.

Eapen, V., Cavanna, A.E., and Robertson, M.M. (2016). Comorbidities, social impact, and quality of life in Tourette's disorder. *Frontiers in Psychiatry* 7: 97. https://doi.org/10.3389/fpsyt.2016.00097.

National Institute for Health and Care Excellence (NICE) (2016). Mental health problems in people with learning disabilities: prevention, assessment and management. NICE guideline [NG54]. https://www.nice.org.uk/guidance/ng54

Young, S., Moss, D., Sedgwick, O. et al. (2015). A meta-analysis of the prevalence of attention deficit hyperactivity disorder in incarcerated populations. *Psychological Medicine* 45 (2): 247–258.

CHAPTER 30

The Genetic Basis of Neurodevelopmental Disorders

F. Lucy Raymond

OVERVIEW

- Global developmental delay, Intellectual disability (ID), autistic spectrum disorder and epilepsy frequently have an underlying genetic cause and in many cases the gene abnormalities that cause the conditions will be the same.

- With the advent of modern genomics, it can be estimated that ~50% of children with moderate to severe ID will have an underlying genetic anomaly.

- De novo variants without a family history are the most frequent cause of disease.

- All children with global developmental delay should be considered for array comparative genomic hybridisation (CGH) testing. Those with a negative result should proceed to more extensive genetic tests with whole-exome or whole-genome sequencing if there is moderate to profound ID.

- Making a diagnosis early can enable further investigation of a child who is vulnerable and needs support and care of both their physical and mental health.

The term neurodevelopmental disorder (NDD) is commonly used as an umbrella term to describe children with a range of features including global developmental delay and intellectual disability/intellectual developmental disorder (ID/IDD), autistic spectrum disorder (ASD), attention deficit hyperactivity disorder (ADHD), developmental coordination disorder and Tourette's. In addition, epilepsy is often considered by some to belong to the same category of disorders, although it is not classified within DSM-5-TR or ICD-11 as such. This chapter will address the genetic basis of NDDs by focusing on global developmental delay/ID and autism.

Historically, in order to identify the genetic basis of each of these conditions, research has focused on ascertaining cohorts of individuals with one phenotypic feature only in order to dissect the underlying aetiology more accurately for each phenotypic trait. While this is an excellent strategy for gene identification and discovery, it has promoted the concept that each of the phenotypes is due to separate and distinct genes. Increasingly, with the advent of modern genomic analysis, this assumption is being challenged, as many of the genes and even specific mutations identified in each cohort are one and the same. An individual with a mutation in any one gene may manifest a combination of epilepsy, ID and/or ASD that is specific to that individual.

Genetic basis of severe intellectual disability

Intelligence quotient (IQ) is defined using a standardised set of test measurements and is predicted to be normally distributed in the population. Within the normal range (<2 standard deviations from the mean) the IQ of a child is strongly predicted from the IQ of both parents. However, at the lower IQ range of <50 there is a significant bulge in the curve, indicating that other aetiological factors account for very low IQ (Figure 30.1).

Also, there is a considerable excess of male children with low IQ, suggesting that X-linked disease may account for some of the increased male preponderance. A key observation is that severe ID is rarely familial, as adults with severe ID tend not to go on to have their own children. This means that if there is a genetic basis to ID there is likely to be either a significant new mutation rate, de novo, which is not sustained in the population, or familial severe ID present in male children may be due to X-linked disease inherited from an unaffected or mildly affected mother.

The unravelling of the genetic basis of ID has only been made possible by the gradual and systematic improvement in methods of genetic analysis. Initially whole-chromosome analysis revealed a few cases of ID due to large microscopically visible deletions or duplications. Ever more detailed analysis of the genetic code to the current fine level of whole-genome analysis, where every base of the genetic code is analysed, has enabled well over 1000 single genes and many microdeletions or duplications to be identified associated with a phenotype of ID.

For some individuals and families, identifying the aetiology of their disorder has clinical value, especially at the extreme end of the spectrum. For some who are at the mildest end of the spectrum, investigating the aetiology of their disorder may be unhelpful as it

ABC of Neurodevelopmental Disorders, First Edition. Edited by Munib Haroon.
© 2024 John Wiley & Sons Ltd. Published 2024 by John Wiley & Sons Ltd.

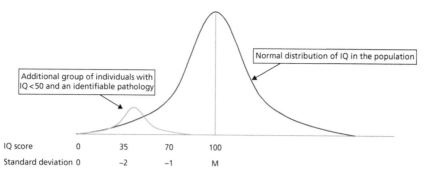

Figure 30.1 IQ distribution in the general population.

is difficult to identify a single genetic cause and this can lead to perceptions of inappropriate labelling. However, in a clinical setting where parents seek information and understanding of their child's condition, especially where the symptoms are severe and are associated with multiple medical problems, this may be a starting point for understanding and potential treatments.

For the group of individuals with moderate to severe ID, there is a >50% chance of finding a genetic change that can be attributed to the condition. For such children presenting to a neurodevelopmental service, it is recommended that testing the genome at low resolution by array comparative genome hybridisation (CGH) is offered. Community paediatricians now use arrays as a first-line investigation for children presenting with delayed development to paediatric services. This is a cheap and comprehensive survey of the whole genetic code, but the resolution is only >100 KB and it will not identify any abnormalities within individual genes, only assessing the genome for large deletions or duplications that are present in the sample. This will account for approximately 10% of cases.

Finding a specific rare copy number variant (CNV) in a child will provide an explanation to parents of why their child has problems (a CNV is a phenomenon in which sequences of the genome are repeated, with the number of repeats varying between individuals). Secondly, it may highlight further testing and assessment needs for the child. The extent of the ID/developmental delay may need further investigation and the genetic change present in the child may be associated with additional clinical features such as epilepsy, growth and feeding difficulties, cardiac and other physical health risks and/or mental health conditions that can be anticipated and monitored.

Rare CNVs within the genome of children with ID or developmental delay are present at many different loci across the whole genome and are associated with ID; many new syndromes are described where ID and ASD coexist. The size and location of the CNV predict the severity to some extent, as does the inheritance pattern. Those CNVs that arise for the first time, de novo, in a child tend to be more associated with severe ID compared to familial CNVs. Indeed, some CNVs, such as 16p11.2 deletion, are fairly common in the general population, although more frequent in the population with mild to moderate ID, some of whom also have ASD.

A subset of rare CNVs in the population are particularly associated with mental health problems and have been extensively studied as individual cohorts. These include 1q21.1 deletion and duplication, 2p16.3 deletion, 9q34.3 deletion, 15q11.2 deletion, 15q13.3

deletion and duplication, 16p11.2 deletion and duplication and 22q11.2 deletion and duplication. In a cohort of 258 individuals with ID and one of these anomalies (Chawner et al. 2019), 80% met the criteria for one or more psychiatric disorders and were impaired across all neurodevelopmental, cognitive and psychopathological traits compared with controls. The risk of ADHD (odds ratio [OR] 6.9, 3.2–15.1), oppositional defiant disorder (OR 3.6, 1.4–9.4), any anxiety disorder (OR 2.9, 1.2–6.7) and ASD traits (OR 44.1, 15.3–127.5) was particularly high compared with controls.

CNVs in children are either inherited from a parent or arise de novo in the child. The behavioural phenotype in children with familial CNV is more marked compared to those with de novo variants, suggesting that the environment of the child and other parentally inherited variants may also contribute significantly to the penetrance of a CNV variant. It appears that children with familial CNVs are especially vulnerable and may benefit from being highlighted for early support and care.

For most CNVs, the exact gene that is responsible for the phenotype is unclear, and the penetrance of the variant (how likely it is to cause the disease) is variable. Rare CNVs are more likely to cause disease than common single nucleotide polymorphisms (SNPs), but less likely than rare single-gene abnormalities.

Initial investigation of a child with ID uses microarray CGH (aCGH) technology. If a negative result is observed, this means either that there is no significant single genomic disorder to be identified or that the aCGH is too blunt an instrument with insufficient resolution to identify single gene abnormalities in the sample. A negative result leads to a binary decision either to do no further testing or to initiate more expensive high-resolution analysis of the genome using gene panels, exome or whole genomes via clinical genetics services.

Factors that will assist in the decision-making tree are how severe the ID is and whether there are additional clinical features (Figure 30.2). Children with mild developmental delay are unlikely to have easily identifiable single-gene disorders and currently are not recommended for further testing, while those with moderate, severe or profound ID should continue to be investigated. As most individuals with severe ID have a single-gene disorder that has arisen de novo, testing samples from both parents alongside the child is invaluable. This trio (parents and child) analysis enables a comparison of the child's DNA with parents and subtraction analysis highlights only those de novo variants in the child that are absent from either parent. Subsequent analysis can assess each of these de novo variants as to whether it is likely to be the cause of disease.

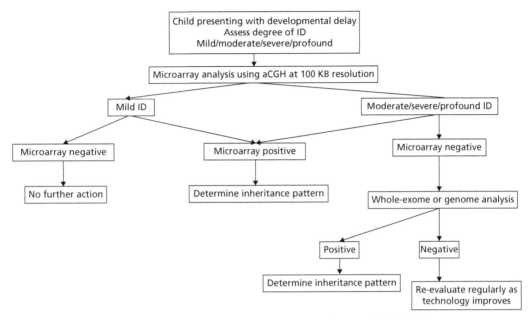

Figure 30.2 Diagnostic decision tree for intellectual disability (ID). aCGH, microarray comparative genomic hybridisation.

If both parents are unavailable to contribute to the analysis, it is intrinsically more limited and a specified panel of genes or list of previously identified variants can only be analysed and reported. This will have a lower diagnostic yield compared to a gene-agnostic approach, but nevertheless will make many more diagnoses than limited analysis by aCGH assessment alone.

Additional features that encourage further genomic analysis if aCGH is negative are the presence of female genomic sex of a child with ID, as these children are more likely to have a genomic disorder. The data shows that a diagnosis of ASD is rarer in females with the same mutation as males. Females show reduced penetrance of a genomic disorder and therefore tend to have a higher mutational burden before manifesting an NDD. The language of the interpretation of this observation is potentially fraught with prejudice. A concept of a female protective model suggesting genomic resilience for females is proposed, but this can also be interpreted as a genomic vulnerability to genomic insults and lack of resilience of the male genotype. What is clear is that there are significant differences between the sexes thought to be due to differences in gene expression in males and females, and that this accounts for the higher prevalence of ID and ASD in males compared to females.

Further additional clinical features are the presence of severe ASD and/or a seizure disorder in children, which is also predictive of a genomic disorder, and these children should be prioritised for extensive genomic investigation. Such children are most likely to have a rare genetic change, but all children with significant (moderate to profound) developmental delay or ID should be considered for testing (see Box 30.1).

Individual rare damaging mutations in specific single genes can be assigned a causative role as the penetrance of the variant is usually high. Identifying single-gene disorders requires detailed sequence analysis of coding genes. Initially, technically limited analysis of the X chromosome identified many rare X-linked

genes that cause ID and ASD. Based on this analysis, a further 1000+ genes were predicted to cause ID and ASD when autosomes were analysed.

Using next-generation sequencing technologies – the ability to sequence whole exomes (the coding part of the genome) or whole genomes at scale – has revolutionised our knowledge of rare genetic events that cause both ID and ASD phenotypes. Large-scale analysis of many families with X-linked disease and subsequently a trio (parents and child) design has been fundamental.

In children with no family history and severe disease, the presence of rare de novo mutational events in synaptic, transcriptional and chromatin genes is increasingly identifiable. For any one individual a single mutational event in any one of thousands of genes is likely to cause disease. In most cases, the phenotypic variation within a child is not easily predictable from the gene that carries the mutation, nor is the phenotype a good predictor of the likely gene that is mutated. This means that historical targeted analysis for a few genes as good candidates for a specific phenotype is clinically misleading and will miss the correct diagnosis if the right gene with a mutation has not been tested. The term 'no abnormality has been detected' perhaps should be replaced with 'insufficient analysis of the genome has been performed'.

Using a gene-agnostic approach to the whole genome or exome has identified many new genes that cause ID and ASD. Analysis of

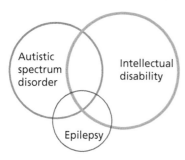

Figure 30.3 Venn diagram illustrating the genomic overlap between intellectual disability, autistic spectrum disorder and epilepsy.

separate cohorts ascertained by meeting ASD criteria or meeting ID criteria reveals a strong overlap in the genes that have been identified. In addition, many genes that have been identified by analysis of cohorts of children with epilepsy also have mutations in many of the same genes involved in ASD and ID. The overlap is not so substantial for ASD and epilepsy, but indicates that rare deleterious mutations in a set of genes can result in a complex array of phenotypes (see Figure 30.3) that include ID, ASD and epilepsy.

Contribution of common genomic variations to autistic spectrum disorder

It has long been recognised from twin studies comparing the rates of ID or autism in monozygotic twins with dizygotic twins that NDDs have a strong genetic predisposition. There is a significant inherited component to autism and many individuals will have other close family members who are either diagnosed with ASD or are affected to a varying degree and who may not quite meet diagnostic criteria. As the name implies, there is a spectrum or continuum of phenotypes that has been recognised within the population, where some individuals meet the diagnostic criteria and others do not. Over the years the number of twins that have been studied has increased, which has enabled a more accurate assessment of the familial component to autism. Meta-analyses of the studies available to date continue to support this early observation. This means that ASD is more likely to be present in close family relatives of someone who has been diagnosed with ASD.

In order to accurately quantify the inherited component of ASD, many studies have been conducted, including one international large-scale study analysing over two million individuals in five countries (Bai et al. 2019). The study measured the extent of the heritable contribution to ASD and found that approximately 80% of the variance in ASD in the population is due to genetic predisposition, with possible modest differences in the sources of ASD risk. This finding has been replicated across countries. What this means in practice is that 80% of the chance of developing ASD is due to an inherited genetic code shared with parents and close relatives, rather than environmental factors, or is due to random mutations found only in the affected individual. These genome-wide association studies (GWASs) analyse DNA from affected and unaffected individuals and look at common variation within the genome that is present in all individuals.

For those variants that are frequent in the general population, no one variant is responsible for autism alone. What matters is the combinations of many variants, each of which could be one of two possible letters (A or T; G or C); this has been the subject of further analysis. The studies look to see if one combination of multiple common variants is more frequent in the affected population compared to the unaffected. GWAS analysis looks at approximately 700 000 SNP variants, each one of which could be one or another version or allele. This provides a huge possible number of combinations, but still only represents <1% of the human genome, although it is focused on the most variable parts. A recent publication (Grove et al. 2019) includes 18 000 cases of autism compared to 28 000 cases without autism and identified several novel genomic loci that are important in conferring the risk, or chance, of developing autism. Only a few of the common variants identified are within the coding region of genes. Most variants are in the non-coding region within or between genes, which does not alter the protein structure of the gene product itself. The effect of the non-coding variants is to alter more subtle regulation of gene expression of the nearby gene in specific tissues. In most cases, how the variant alters expression is not clearly identified but is assumed; which tissues are critical is unknown.

Large-scale association studies can be used to generate a polygenic risk score (PRS) that has the potential to be used to assess an individual's risk of developing ASD compared to individuals not on the autistic spectrum. This, however, estimates a relative risk, as it compares groups with a certain disorder and those without the disorder. Also, it requires one to know which genes and variants are associated with the condition, which for autism is still far from entirely clear at this stage. Furthermore, PRSs compare like with like and as most studies to date are in the Caucasian population, this type of scoring is only valid within the Caucasian population. Nevertheless, there are huge research resources invested to understand which variations in the genome are important contributors to autistic behaviours as a first step to understanding the neurobiological process involved in this complex disorder.

It appears that the phenotypic manifestation of ASD in an individual is a combined effect of rare variants, both from very rare or unique de novo variants in single genes, rare CNVs and also multiple common SNPs contributing to the person's polygenic risk scores, as well as the sex of the child (Figure 30.4). The effect of a rare variant is likely to be context dependent. In children with a high polygenic predisposition to ASD who also have a rare deleterious mutation, the likelihood of manifesting an ASD phenotype is far higher than in the context of a low polygenic predisposition (Figure 30.5). In a high-risk individual who has inherited a significant number of risk-contributing SNPs, the addition of a rare deleterious mutation may be more likely to lead to an autism phenotype than in a low-risk individual.

Due to resource constraints within the NHS, further detailed genetic investigation of the genome will need to be limited to children with the most severe ASD and those who have additional features, including significant developmental delay or epilepsy. In these cases, either limited targeted analysis or whole-genome sequence analysis should be offered to identify the cause. In a few years, full trio genome sequencing will be available to all those children presenting with ASD or ID. This means that there continue to be some

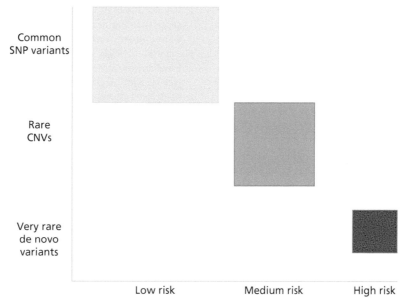

Figure 30.4 Both very rare and more common variants contribute to autism spectrum disorder. CNV, copy number variant; SNP, single-nucleotide polymorphism.

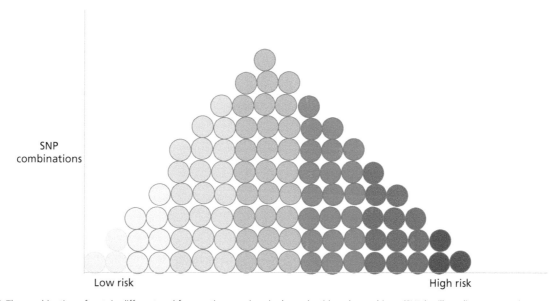

Figure 30.5 The combination of certain different and frequently occurring single-nucleotide polymorphisms (SNPs) will predispose to autism spectrum disorder more than other combinations.

children without a genomic diagnosis due to lack of technology and availability. Currently, the inability to identify a genetic cause of disease in a child is more likely to be due to the failure of genetic investigation than the assumption that 'it's not genetic', which was so often suggested in the past. The science of interrogating the genome fully still has a long way to go to identify all rare variations.

Conclusion

This chapter has focused on the genetic variation that underlies ID, global developmental delay and ASD, and just as our understanding of the genetic aetiology for these conditions continues to develop, the same may be said for other NDDs. But genetic aetiology needs to be put in context. For example, evidence presented elsewhere in this book clearly indicates the critical importance of a person's environment in manifesting NDDs. The data indicates that poor social circumstances, traumatic experiences and exposure to environmental substances (whether in utero or ex utero) are critical aetiological factors that need to be assessed alongside the genetic components of these complex conditions.

Further reading

Antaki, D., Guevara, J., Maihofer, A.X. et al. (2022). A phenotypic spectrum of autism is attributable to the combined effects of rare variants, polygenic risk and sex. *Nature Genetics* 54 (9): 1284–1292.

Bai, D., Yip, B.H.K., Windham, G.C. et al. (2019). Association of genetic and environmental factors with autism in a 5-country cohort. *JAMA Psychiatry* 76 (10): 1035–1043.

Bailey, A., Le Couteur, A., Gottesman, I. et al. (1995). Autism as a strongly genetic disorder: evidence from a British twin study. *Psychological Medicine* 25 (1): 63–77.

Chawner, S., Owen, M.J., Holmans, P. et al. (2019). Genotype–phenotype associations in children with copy number variants associated with high neuropsychiatric risk in the UK (IMAGINE-ID): a case–control cohort study. *Lancet Psychiatry* 6 (6): 493–505.

Colvert, E., Tick, B., McEwen, F. et al. (2015). Heritability of autism spectrum disorder in a UK population-based twin sample. *JAMA Psychiatry* 72 (5): 415–423.

Cooper, G.M., Coe, B.P., Girirajan, S. et al. (2011). A copy number variation morbidity map of developmental delay. *Nature Genetics* 43 (9): 838–846.

De Rubeis, S., He, X., Goldberg, A.P. et al. (2014). Synaptic, transcriptional and chromatin genes disrupted in autism. *Nature* 515 (7526): 209–215.

Deciphering Developmental Disorders Study (2017). Prevalence and architecture of de novo mutations in developmental disorders. *Nature* 542 (7642): 433–438.

Epi, K.C. (2012). Epi4K: gene discovery in 4,000 genomes. *Epilepsia* 53 (8): 1457–1467.

Epi4K Consortium, Epilepsy Phenome/Genome Project, Allen, A.S., Berkovic, S.F. et al. (2013). De novo mutations in epileptic encephalopathies. *Nature* 501 (7466): 217–221.

Grove, J., Ripke, S., Als, T.D. et al. (2019). Identification of common genetic risk variants for autism spectrum disorder. *Nature Genetics* 51 (3): 431–444.

Iossifov, I., O'Roak, B.J., Sanders, S.J. et al. (2014). The contribution of de novo coding mutations to autism spectrum disorder. *Nature* 515 (7526): 216–221.

Jacquemont, S., Coe, B.P., Hersch, M. et al. (2014). A higher mutational burden in females supports a 'female protective model' in neurodevelopmental disorders. *American Journal of Human Genetics* 94 (3): 415–425.

Jamain, S., Quach, H., Betancur, C. et al. (2003). Mutations of the X-linked genes encoding neuroligins NLGN3 and NLGN4 are associated with autism. *Nature Genetics* 34 (1): 27–29.

Malinowski, J., Miller, D.T., Demmer, L. et al. (2020). Systematic evidence-based review: outcomes from exome and genome sequencing for pediatric patients with congenital anomalies or intellectual disability. *Genetics in Medicine* 22 (6): 986–1004.

Neale, B.M., Kou, Y., Liu, L. et al. (2012). Patterns and rates of exonic de novo mutations in autism spectrum disorders. *Nature* 485 (7397): 242–245.

Rolland, T., Cliquet, F., Anney, R.J.L. et al. (2023). Phenotypic effects of genetic variants associated with autism. *Nature Medicine* 29: 1671–1680.

Schneider, M., Debbane, M., Bassett, A.S. et al. (2014). Psychiatric disorders from childhood to adulthood in 22q11.2 deletion syndrome: results from the International Consortium on Brain and Behavior in 22q11.2 deletion syndrome. *American Journal of Psychiatry* 171 (6): 627–639.

Tarpey, P.S., Smith, R., Pleasance, E. et al. (2009). A systematic, large-scale resequencing screen of X-chromosome coding exons in mental retardation. *Nature Genetics* 41 (5): 535–543.

Taylor, M.J., Rosenqvist, M.A., Larsson, H. et al. (2020). Etiology of autism spectrum disorders and autistic traits over time. *JAMA Psychiatry* 77 (9): 936–943.

Thompson, L.A., Detterman, D.K., and Plomin, R. (1993). Differences in heritability across groups differing in ability, revisited. *Behavior Genetics* 23 (4): 331–336.

Tick, B., Bolton, P., Happe, F. et al. (2016). Heritability of autism spectrum disorders: a meta-analysis of twin studies. *Journal of Child Psychology and Psychiatry* 57 (5): 585–595.

Wolstencroft, J., Wicks, F., Srinivasan, R. et al. (2022). Neuropsychiatric risk in children with intellectual disability of genetic origin: IMAGINE, a UK national cohort study. *Lancet Psychiatry* 9 (9): 715–724.

CHAPTER 31

Neurodivergency on a Day-to-Day Basis

Munib Haroon

Neurodivergency is common. Taken as a whole, these conditions are present in 15–20% of the population. So it is not just your patients: you, your partner, child, father, mother, sibling, colleague, line manager or subordinate may be neurodivergent. But not everyone who is neurodivergent ends up with a clinical diagnosis. There will be many reasons for this and people will be in a number of potentially different situations (Box 31.1). As such, the clinical presentation of neurodivergency and of neurodevelopmental disorders is probably the tip of the iceberg (Figure 31.1).

For many people, the lived experience of being different will be one that does not involve seeking a diagnosis. Despite this, there can often be a combination of challenges in navigating a way through childhood and into adulthood. This may be because of functional difficulties, which may be intrinsic to the condition or entirely due to the environment, or a combination of the two; it may be down to societal issues. Although neurodiversity is an increasingly understood and accepted phenomenon, those who are neurodivergent still face marginalisation and discrimination, and the stigma around the condition may be one of the reasons that people do not seek a diagnosis.

There is much that can be done to support the neurodivergent in different environments. This chapter offers up some very broad themes for support, including thoughts from individuals who are neurodivergent (Boxes 31.2 and 31.3).

Difference can require a different approach

In many walks of life, like at school and at work, getting everyone to work in the same way (reducing variation is a fundamental approach to project management methodologies like Six Sigma) can be good to ensure consistency. However, many of the day-to-day institutions we rely on are largely made up *of*, *by* and *for* neurotypical people, and so may not be optimised to do things for those who think, perceive and function differently. So whether you teach a 7-year-old school boy or train a 30-year-old doctor, it is important to think about those who think differently.

Dealing with the person not the label

While it is crucial to be aware of diagnostic labels and try to proceed accordingly, there is such breadth in the presentation of neurodivergency that it is important to avoid adopting a stereotypical attitude. In addition, not everyone has a diagnosis, or will be ready to offer it up. If it is felt that someone needs a particular intervention, then starting a discussion around what it is thought may be helpful for them as opposed to trying to have a discussion about diagnoses may be a better start.

Being environmentally aware

The environment around a person has a great effect on how well they can manage. How well would anyone manage with their day-to-day tasks if they were parachuted into the middle of the Amazon rainforest? There are many aspects of a person's environment to consider. This can be their inorganic environment, such as surrounding materials, noises or temperature, or it can be related to

ABC of Neurodevelopmental Disorders, First Edition. Edited by Munib Haroon.
© 2024 John Wiley & Sons Ltd. Published 2024 by John Wiley & Sons Ltd.

Figure 31.1 The clinical presentation of neurodivergency and of neurodevelopmental disorders is probably the tip of the iceberg.

people – the scent of sandwiches, the chatter of conversation or having someone intruding on your personal space.

No man is an island

Personal networks are also very important. It is important to see people in relation to others, whether this is as part of a family, classroom or organisation. These domains are themselves nested within

a wider societal context. Such networks have an influence on the neurodivergent and vice versa (Figure 31.2).

Strengths

Being neurodivergent comes with many strengths. People who are neurodivergent may be able to focus for long periods of time on specific issues long after others have gotten tired, they may have an eye for detail, they may think differently and thus help reduce groupthink in an organisation. To get to where they want to go they will invariably have to show a considerable degree of tenacity.

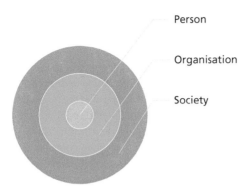

Person

Organisation

Society

Figure 31.2 No man is an island. Personal networks are important. It is important to see people in relation to others, whether this is as part of a family, classroom or organisation.

Think about the comorbidities

It is important to remember that it may not be a diagnosed neurodevelopmental condition that is causing a person difficulties. It may be a comorbid condition that has been hitherto undiagnosed.

The law

The law underpins a lot of what can be done to help neurodivergent people on a day-to-day basis. In the United Kingdom, this includes human rights legislation. This is enshrined in the Human Rights Act 1998 and the Equality Act 2010, the latter designed to protect people (including those with a disability) from discrimination in the workplace and wider society. An underlying principle of all these provisions is the right to human dignity. Additionally, the Autism Act 2009, the first disability-specific piece of legislation, places a statutory duty on the NHS and local authorities to provide appropriate services to assess autism in adults and to support them post diagnosis. This was followed in 2021 with a national strategy for children, young people and adults with autism, with a broad remit to improve their outcomes.

The law is always changing, but it is also fair to say that the law changes slowly, reactively and is open to interpretation. Not only does the law state what can and cannot be done, but it – via the courts – also acts as the arbiter of last resort for many disputes. Hence there is the potential for improvements to the situation of neurodivergent people to be achieved via litigation. However, accessing the mechanisms that allow for this to take place relies on knowing when and where and from whom to seek appropriate advice and information. Despite many free (and paid) resources and services offering information and support, the time and effort required to 'take legal action', navigating a way through the procedures and paperwork, can prove to be a barrier for some.

School

For children deemed to have special educational needs (SEN) and disabilities (which will include many children and young people with a feature of a neurodevelopmental condition) there are two broad levels of support at school: SEN support and a formalised Education, Health and Care plan (EHCP). Within this framework there are many adjustments and supportive processes that can be put into place according to the individual needs of the child. (Some examples are shown in Box 31.4.)

Box 31.4 John and school

John, 10 years old, has autism and an intellectual disability. He had been behind his peers at school for a number of years, requiring one-to-one support for much of the day and supervision during break times as well as communication support. The classroom environment was modified to take his sensory needs into account and he was allowed to wear noise defenders in the classroom, as well as having adaptations to his school uniform. Simple adjustments like always being first in line and being allowed to focus on his love of numbers also helped.

Initially his school considered that the SEN support he was receiving was sufficient; despite this, his family felt that he was falling behind and was in need of additional support. The family felt that an EHCP was required and asked the local authority to carry this out. The local authority decided against this, on the basis that everything that needed to be done was already being done. The family challenged the decision, appealing to the SEN and Disability Tribunal, which decided against the local authority's decision. The local authority carried out an assessment and John was issued with an EHCP. He now attends a special school and because of challenging behaviours he also receives free transport to school.

The key to providing appropriately tailored support is ongoing monitoring of the child's needs, making adjustments, seeing their effect and making further changes as required. Clear communication between carers and the school about what is being done, what is required and what the family can do if they are not happy with what is being done is important.

For many children a mainstream setting works best, although this may not be full time, while for others a special school setting is preferable. There are options in between the two and there can also be the option of home schooling. While school can be challenging at times for everyone, it can be particularly challenging for those who are neurodivergent and the memories of such times can cast a long shadow, as can academic underperformance (see Box 31.5).

Work

An employment gap exists for neurodiverse people, meaning that they are likely to have poorer employment outcomes compared to the general population. Data from the UK's Office for National Statistics for 2021 shows that people with severe or specific learning difficulties had the lowest employment rates (26%), followed by individuals with autism (29%), followed by those with mental illness or other nervous disorders (30.1%).

One of the relevant key pieces of legislation in the Equality Act relates to reasonable adjustments that employers must make for workers with disabilities or physical or mental health conditions so that they are not substantially disadvantaged when doing their jobs. A formal diagnosis is not required to request such adjustments, but an employer could decline such requests if they do not deem a person to have a disability, in the absence of a diagnosis. In such circumstances dispute resolution or grievance procedures may need to be instigated. Additionally, there are schemes in the UK such as Access to Work, a publicly funded programme that can help neurodivergent people to start or stay in work. This may be by financing

Box 31.5 **M on school**

'School was possibly the biggest challenge I've faced in my entire life. I have done a lot of things since, I have more letters after my name than within my actual name, but I'd single out my school days (the best days of our lives!) as the time that I was on the knife-edge of possibility. I stood out. I had a different accent. My fashion sense was different to other boys – driven largely by the idiosyncratic costume choices of the BBC when choosing the wardrobes for their Dr Whos. This tended to me make me a bit of a bully magnet, which was exacerbated by periods where I tended to retreat into my own shell. I was slow to make friends. I was very encyclopaedic in some interests, yes, *The Little Professor*, but I was often so distracted by what was going on in my head that entire lessons could pass me by and I'd scramble to work out what I was supposed to be doing by looking at what the child next to me was writing. I loved a lot of sports but this wasn't helped by my terrible ball skills. Kicking and throwing was fine as long as it wasn't in a straight line – although a long summer of intense practice, to the amazement of my friends, seemed to do the trick. I was terrible with homework – I'd often forget, or do it last minute or just not see the point of why it was important. Important letters stayed in my bag all week. In the end, I overcame a lot of this by sheer hard work (as well as focusing on the subjects that I had a great aptitude for). But I'd have benefited from a lot more enthusiasm from teachers when it came to topics I was interested in (when I wanted to know what electricity was at 10, or what calculus was at 12, I remember being fobbed off and told to wait until it was the right time! What? Then *was* the right time!). This was before the internet, there were no mobile phones to serve up everything on a plate.

I grew up in a very different era, and what would have been most useful was more knowledge about why I was different – I wasn't difficult or bad or lazy. I know things have changed, but not enough, in my opinion. Bullying at primary and middle school made a *huge* difference to my learning (and I'm not just talking about pupils) and I'm sure I spent large periods of time worrying and anxious, and this resulted in a huge amount of time off school. I estimate that my attendance pre-high school (<13) was around 80–90%. Taking up karate helped my self-esteem and once I could show I wasn't a pushover things got better, but I wish teachers were better at nipping things in the bud, or were always part of the solution as opposed to, on one occasion, the actual problem.

So. . . Different or disordered? In my case it was both, I can't see how having attention deficit was anything but the greatest of impediments to doing anything, but many of my other differences go to the heart of me, or perhaps I should say that they go to the very neurons of me, and I would not change them for the world. I see patterns. I see connections. I see things in the sea of life that others don't seem to see.

Were my difficulties innate or environmental? I think there was an element of both.

Everyone has a different story to tell, but if I remind *you* of yourself, what I'd say is this: Back yourself 100%. Don't let others' underestimation of you weigh you down. Don't stand for bullying. Work out what works for you in learning and in life, and do it quickly, and get others to help you. Play to your strengths, but don't neglect weaker areas. Try to find peace in your difference: it can be a great gift, albeit one that is difficult to unwrap.'

a grant to pay for a job coach or for car adaptations or to provide one-to-one mental health sessions. It does not fund reasonable adjustments.

Yet neurodiverse people have undoubtedly made great contributions to art and science despite remaining under-represented in the workplace. One area where the strength of the neurodivergent (specifically those who are autistic) is well recognised is in the field of computer science/programming and information technology. Box 31.6 shows a case study of how one company in Poland, the asperIT Foundation, is helping to recruit people with autism into industry, where they can apply their considerable strengths/talents.

The employment gap represents a triple loss: a loss to the neurodivergent individual – and their financial and physical/mental well-being; a loss to the company, which could benefit from the strengths that such individuals bring; and lastly, a loss to wider society. There is also a moral/ethical/legal dimension to this as well as a financial one and much that organisations could do throughout the working life of an individual.

This begins with giving consideration to the job advert and job description, processes at interview, onboarding, time during the job, annual management review and post-employment processes – such as an exit interview that aims to investigate the reasons an employee has left – so that any potential improvements can be made to help with retaining valuable employees (see Figure 31.3).

Box 31.6 **asperIT**

One example of a company that is working to make a difference to the employed lives of the neurodivergent is the asperIT Foundation. Based in Wroclaw, Poland, the foundation supports autistic people to develop competencies that can help them to thrive in IT/computing and other data-focused professions. Recognising the skills that many autistic people have (such as a propensity for attention to detail, excellent pattern recognition, not being as phased by repetition, unlike neurotypicals, perseverance, and an interest in computing), asperIT provides technical support/training while helping with the development of social skills and professional contacts. Much of the training happens during paid internships/apprenticeships with companies that recognise the strengths of a diverse workplace. During/after these placements there is the opportunity to further test these skills in a working environment and potentially find employment with a company that recognises and values them as individuals, while continuing to be mentored and offered support.

As strong advocates for autistic people, asperIT waves the flag for the skills and strengths that neurodivergency can bring to the workplace through a number of other different initiatives, such as delivering workshops and training for HR/recruitment personnel across Poland, raising awareness among universities, and trying to develop a reliable database of information that can be used by other employers to create a friendly working environment for the neurodiverse.

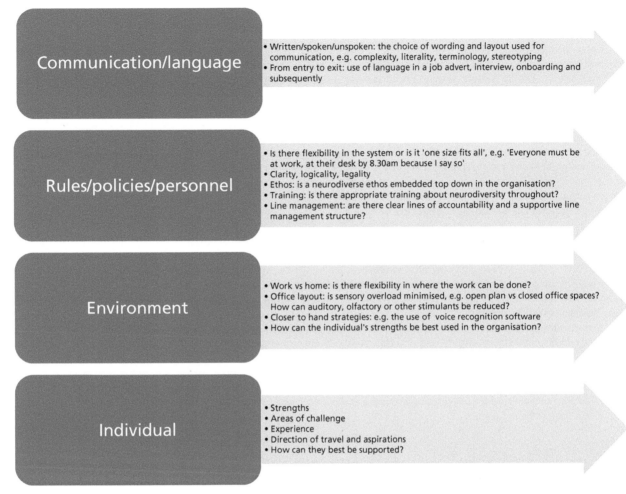

Communication/language
- Written/spoken/unspoken: the choice of wording and layout used for communication, e.g. complexity, literality, terminology, stereotyping
- From entry to exit: use of language in a job advert, interview, onboarding and subsequently

Rules/policies/personnel
- Is there flexibility in the system or is it 'one size fits all', e.g. 'Everyone must be at work, at their desk by 8.30am because I say so'
- Clarity, logicality, legality
- Ethos: is a neurodiverse ethos embedded top down in the organisation?
- Training: is there appropriate training about neurodiversity throughout?
- Line management: are there clear lines of accountability and a supportive line management structure?

Environment
- Work vs home: is there flexibility in where the work can be done?
- Office layout: is sensory overload minimised, e.g. open plan vs closed office spaces? How can auditory, olfactory or other stimulants be reduced?
- Closer to hand strategies: e.g. the use of voice recognition software
- How can the individual's strengths be best used in the organisation?

Individual
- Strengths
- Areas of challenge
- Experience
- Direction of travel and aspirations
- How can they best be supported?

Figure 31.3 Adjustment and adaptations at work. There are different types of adaptations that can be carried out in a work environment to help a neurodivergent individual.

Housing

Neurodivergent people can live in a variety of settings, and while many will live alone or with their families/partners or friends, a small proportion will also live in a registered care home, in sheltered housing or in supported housing/living or shared living schemes. Some adults may not be happy with their living arrangements, especially if they are unable to live as independently as they would like. There can be a number of barriers preventing this, including a mismatch between the supply of appropriate housing and demand, and a lack of information, support and advocacy for families and individuals. Things can be particularly challenging for those individuals with the profoundest level of difficulties, those with behaviours which challenge and those who live with elderly parents. It is important for individuals to have access to advocacy, information and support to make decisions and to plan for the future.

Relationships

All relationships have their moments, the good and the bad; this is as true for relationships involving neurodivergent individuals as it is for their neurotypical counterparts. However, the issues encountered in relationships where one person is neurodivergent can be of a different nature to those in neurotypical relationships.

Some issues are managed with or without difficulty, some require outside support, and some may be the slow-burning fuse that triggers an eventual referral for a diagnostic assessment. Neurodivergent individuals can be parents, children, siblings, partners or friends. Given the hereditary nature of these conditions, the conditions may cluster within a family. On the one hand, having two or more individuals with the same way of thinking and behaving may be helpful, but this may not always be the case; this will be affected by other aspects to do with individual personality, wider social and familial factors, the nature of the condition, its severity, the presence of other medical issues, and the degree of knowledge and insight that people have of their conditions and of themselves. For example, a parent with ADHD may be very attuned to the needs of a child with ADHD, but alternatively they may have such severe inattention that they do not pay much heed to such needs.

This is not a relationship counselling textbook, but many of the foundational principles behind practising good medicine apply to relationships: having a good knowledge base, being reflective, continuing to try to develop oneself, good communication and honesty.

Box 31.7 **N on their neurodivergent partner**

'When I met my partner, it wasn't obvious that he was neurodivergent. I guess that just shows that people who are neurodivergent don't wear a label on their forehead saying so. It also demonstrates that as an adult you can adapt and learn ways of managing aspects of your neurodivergency to make it less noticeable (irrespective of whether that is a good or a bad thing).

However, over the years my partner's autism and ADHD have become more pronounced. I wonder in part if that's related to age. Noticeably, after an episode of Covid-19 I think his neurodivergency came to the fore for six months or so. It may also be because he's more comfortable in not hiding his neurodivergent traits as society starts to recognise and understand neurodiversity a bit more, which I think is a good thing.

I won't lie, having a partner who is neurodivergent is a challenge for me as much as it is for him. He has this brilliant mind and attention to detail for the things he likes or is interested in. But if it's something he doesn't want to do, then he won't do it – period. He also has episodes of flitting continuously from one thing to another, which can be exhausting to watch let alone for him to sustain. He lacks any common sense to the extent that sometimes it's like having a child in the house as opposed to an adult partner. And he is not at all good with emotion. If I get upset, I don't get a receptive response, in fact it simply makes him annoyed and uncomfortable.

But when on point, and riding high with hyperactivity, he achieves so much for himself and so well. His strong sense of advocacy and justice is admirable.

He likes routine, which is fine because I do too, but I need to be careful when requesting that he does some tasks. Too many in one go just leads to overload and nothing being done. Better to explain one task, get it done and then move on to the next if I want a productive outcome for my 'Wish List'. As I've said, if he's not interested in something – and usually that's the mundaneness of running a house – then he won't do it or see the point in doing something, so he doesn't remember what to do. A list is then a good reminder.

It's important for me to remember my husband is my partner, I'm not his carer or his pseudo-parent. It's unhelpful to him to take over his life in that way, disempowering him and creating an unequal balance in the relationship.

I have to mention food. I'm probably the world's worst cook. But that's ok because his tastes are simple, he likes the same things over and over again, and he's uncomplaining about what he gets on a plate. It's about routine and consistency for him. But he also reminds me not to sweat about the small things in life, which I'm otherwise prone to do.

I'm not the most patient of people so I've had to cultivate that over the years in response to my partner. But that's a good thing. So, I guess what I am saying is that neurodivergent people can change those around them for the positive. It's easy to be distracted by some of the challenges, but instead there's lots of positives to come out of a relationship in which someone is neurodivergent and which remind you why you fell in love with them in the first place.'

It is important to state that relationships matter to all neurodivergent people and that relationships are good for well being in general. Common stereotypes such as 'individuals with autism are loners and introverts' may capture *some* of the nature of the condition for some people while also being highly misleading caricatures.

What can be said for all human beings can be said for neurodivergent people: relationships require nurture, and when things are not going right, it is important to think about the wider determinants of what makes a relationship tick. It is important to remember that relationships are two-way dynamic processes and to keep in mind what is most valuable about them (Box 31.7). It can be unhelpful for one person in a relationship to pin the blame for everything on the neurodivergent person or their condition. It is important to know when to seek outside help and to know that doing so is not a sign of inadequacy.

Further reading

Office for National Statistics (2022). Outcomes for disabled people in the UK: 2021. https://www.ons.gov.uk/peoplepopulationandcommunity/health andsocialcare/disability/articles/outcomesfordisabledpeopleintheuk/2021

Smith, T. and Kirby, A. (2021). *Neurodiversity at Work*. London: Kogan Page.

Index

Note: *Italic* page numbers refer to figure and **Bold** page numbers reference to tables.

ABC of Neurodevelopmental Disorders, First Edition. Edited by Munib Haroon.

© 2024 John Wiley & Sons Ltd. Published 2024 by John Wiley & Sons Ltd.